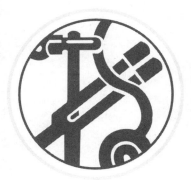

Student Workbook for
Mosby's Guide to Physical Examination

Fifth Edition

Henry M. Seidel, MD
Professor Emeritus of Pediatrics
The Johns Hopkins University School of Medicine
Baltimore, Maryland

Jane W. Ball, RN, DrPH, CPNP
Director, Emergency Medical Services for Children
National Resource Center
Children's National Medical Center
Washington, DC

Joyce E. Dains, DrPH, JD, RN, CS, FNP
Assistant Professor
Department of Family and Community Medicine
Baylor College of Medicine
Houston, Texas

G. William Benedict, MD, PhD
Assistant Professor, Medicine
The Johns Hopkins University School of Medicine
Baltimore, Maryland

Prepared by

Linda Lea Kerby, RNC, BSN, MA
Mastery Educational Consultations
Leawood, Kansas

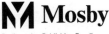 **Mosby**
Dedicated to Publishing Excellence

Mosby, Inc.
An Imprint of Elsevier Science
St. Louis   London   Philadelphia   Sydney   Toronto

D1472247

Vice President and Publishing Director: Sally Schrefer
Managing Editor: Lee Henderson

NOTICE

Health care is an ever-changing field. Standard safety precautions must be followed, but as new research and clinical experience broaden our knowledge, changes in treatment and drug therapy may become necessary or appropriate. Readers are advised to check the most current product information provided by the manufacturer of each drug to be administered to verify the recommended dose, the method and duration of administration, and contraindications. It is the responsibility of the licensed prescriber, relying on experience and knowledge of the patient, to determine dosages and the best treatment for each individual patient. Neither the Publisher nor the editor assume any liability for any injury and/ or damage to persons or property arising from this publication

The Publisher

Copyright © 2003, 1999, 1995, 1991, 1987, Mosby, Inc. All rights reserved.

No part of this publication may be reproduced or transmitted in any form or by any means, electronic or mechanical, including photocopy, recording, or any information storage and retrieval system, without permission in writing from the publisher.

Although for mechanical reasons all pages of this publication are perforated, only those pages imprinted with a Mosby, Inc. copyright notice are intended for removal.

Mosby, Inc.
An Imprint of Elsevier Science
11830 Westline Industrial Drive
St. Louis, Missouri 63146

Printed in the United States of America.

Library of Congress Cataloging in Publication Data

International Standard Book Number: 0-323-01675-8

PREFACE

This *Student Workbook* to accompany *Mosby's Guide to Physical Examination*, Fifth Edition, has been designed to help you achieve the goals associated with learning to interview patients for a health history and perform a physical examination. Each chapter in the workbook corresponds to one in the textbook, with the same title and chapter number. The correct answers to the questions are listed in the back of the workbook so that you can evaluate your comprehension of the material.

Each chapter in the workbook begins with a list of Learning Objectives to be used in assessing your comprehension of the material. A variety of exercises in each chapter help you practice and confirm your understanding of the concepts, key terms, and techniques of examination. These exercises include:

- Content Review Questions: Crossword puzzles and questions with multiple choice, fill-in-the-blank, and matching answers will help you review the primary concepts and terminology related to the content. Anatomic drawings to be labeled will challenge you to apply knowledge associated with the relevant body system.
- Concepts Application: Exercises to help you evaluate and assess examination findings to interpret the results and recognize normal and abnormal outcomes.
- Case Study: Case studies give you the opportunity to apply data evaluation skills in a clinical setting. Additional information or data needed to further determine a diagnosis or course of action may be called for, and you will have the opportunity to suggest further examination.
- Critical Thinking: Problems are posed to give you practice in analyzing patient information and managing interactions with patients.

It is my hope that the Workbook will be helpful to you in your study of physical examination. Special thanks to Jean Foret Giddens for her valuable work on previous editions of this workbook, and to Lee Henderson for his continued editorial support and feedback .

Linda Lea Kerby, RNC, BSN, MA
Leawood, Kansas

CONTENTS

The History and Interviewing Process

LEARNING OBJECTIVES

After studying Chapter 1 in the textbook and completing this section of the workbook, students should be able to:

1. Recognize ethical considerations in patient-examiner relationships.
2. Identify aspects of communication that affect the interview process.
3. Describe techniques to facilitate an interview.
4. Discuss elements to include in a history.
5. Organize data according to a clinical history outline.
6. Revise history taking to accommodate variations in age and condition.

TEXTBOOK REVIEW

Chapter 1 The History and Interviewing Process (pages 1–37)

CONTENT REVIEW QUESTIONS

Multiple Choice

Circle the correct answer for each of the following questions.

1. Which of the following will best facilitate the interview when obtaining a history on a deaf patient who can read lips?
   a. speaking loudly
   b. using gestures
   c. speaking slowly
   d. sitting to the side of the patient

Copyright © 2003, Mosby, Inc. All rights reserved.

2. Approximately what percentage of patients interviewed have a sexual orientation other than heterosexual?
   a. 2%
   b. 5%
   c. 10%
   d. 20%

3. During a history, the patient indicates he has an uncle and a brother with sickle cell disease. Which of the following is an appropriate method to document this information?
   a. Document this as chief complaint.
   b. Draw a pedigree diagram.
   c. Include this in past medical history.
   d. Incorporate this information in the social history.

4. Which approach is recommended at the onset of an interview?
   a. Use a structured approach to ask the questions.
   b. Introduce yourself and include a detailed description of your background and qualifications.
   c. Use an open-ended approach; let the patient explain the problem or reason for the visit.
   d. Start with the family history and past medical history to determine the underlying problem.

5. Which of the following questions may lead to an inaccurate patient response?
   a. "Where do you feel the pain?"
   b. "How does this situation make you feel?"
   c. "What happened after you noticed your injury?"
   d. "That was a horrible experience, wasn't it?"

6. Repeating a patient's answer is an attempt to:
   a. confirm an accurate understanding.
   b. discourage patient anger or hostility.
   c. teach the patient new medical terms.
   d. test the patient's knowledge.

7. Which of the following information is unique to a pediatric history?
   a. family history
   b. developmental history
   c. social history
   d. past medical history

8. When interviewing an adolescent patient who is reluctant to talk during an interview, it is best to:
   a. tell the patient you must have straight answers to your questions.
   b. ensure confidentiality regarding information discussed.
   c. inform the patient that adolescents have trouble expressing their feelings.
   d. obtain the history from a parent or other family member.

9. During an interview, your patient admits to feeling worthless and having a sleep disturbance for the last 3 weeks. These are clues that warrant the exploration of:
   a. suicide.
   b. split personality.
   c. cognitive function.
   d. functional assessment.

Copyright © 2003, Mosby, Inc. All rights reserved.

10. Mrs. Carol Turner, a 38-year-old female, brings her 1-year-old son in for health care. Which of the following requests made by the interviewer to the child's mother would be most appropriate at the beginning of an interview?
    a. "Mom, please place your son in your lap."
    b. "Carol, please place your son in your lap."
    c. "Mrs. Turner, please place your son in your lap."
    d. "Sweetie, please place your son in your lap."

11. Which type of questionnaire concerning drug and/or alcohol use is advocated, though not clinically validated, for adolescent patients?
    a. TACE
    b. CAGE
    c. RAFFT
    d. DDST

12. Jerry, a 26-year-old homosexual male, is having a health history taken. Which question regarding sexual activity would most likely *hamper* trust between Jerry and the interviewer?
    a. "Are you married or do you have a girlfriend?"
    b. "Tell me about your living situation."
    c. "Are you sexually active?"
    d. "Are your partners men, women, or both?"

13. A conversation with a parent concerning a 5-year-old child:
    a. violates the child's need for privacy.
    b. is inappropriate since the child is able to talk with you.
    c. provides significant information about family dynamics.
    d. causes distrust in the child toward the examiner.

14. You are interviewing a patient who annoys you and who makes you angry enough that you begin to dislike the patient. The best way to resolve this is to:
    a. use techniques to make the patient like you more.
    b. displace your annoyance towards the patient on an inanimate object.
    c. ignore the feelings and remain neutral in your interactions.
    d. express concern over the situation and explore the problem with the patient.

15. Long periods of silence during an interview may indicate:
    a. a need for the health care provider to increase the pace of the interview.
    b. an inability of the patient to communicate.
    c. a reluctance of the patient to verbalize information.
    d. a need to terminate the interview because of a decreased attention of the patient.

16. Which of the following behaviors describe *intelligent repose*?
    a. Data from the history is documented using direct patient quotes.
    b. Questions are phrased so that they are clear and explicit.
    c. The interviewer avoids the trap of giving advice during an interview.
    d. The interviewer listens intently and observes nonverbal cues.

17. When questioning a patient regarding a sensitive issue such as drug use, it is best to:
    a. begin by describing to the patient the effects of drug abuse on health.
    b. be direct, firm, and to the point.
    c. explain that the information will be shared only by health care workers.
    d. apologize to the patient for asking personal questions.

Copyright © 2003, Mosby, Inc. All rights reserved.

18. Direct questions are designed to:
    a. attack sensitive material head on.
    b. demonstrate to the patient who is in charge of the interview process.
    c. ensure confidentiality.
    d. obtain or clarify specific details about an answer.

19. Interviewers should identify and assess their own feelings, such as hostility and prejudice, in order to:
    a. avoid inappropriate behavior.
    b. explain their biases to patients.
    c. express their idiosyncrasies.
    d. present an integrated persona to the patient.

20. During an interview, a patient describes abdominal pain that often awakens him at night. Which of the following responses by the interviewer would facilitate the interviewing process?
    a. "Constipation can cause abdominal pain."
    b. "Do you need a sleeping medication?"
    c. "Pain is always worse at night, isn't it?"
    d. "Tell me what you mean by 'often.'"

21. When taking a patient's history, you are asked questions about your personal life. What is the best response to facilitate the interviewing process?
    a. Answer briefly and then refocus to the patient's history.
    b. Give as much detail as possible about the asked information.
    c. Ignore the question and continue with the patient's history.
    d. Tell the patient that it is inappropriate to answer personal questions.

22. During an interview, the patient describes problems associated with an illness and begins to cry. The best action in this situation is to:
    a. stop the interview and reschedule for another time.
    b. allow the patient to cry, then resume when the patient is ready.
    c. change the topic to something less upsetting.
    d. continue the interview while the patient cries in order to get through it quickly.

Terminology Review

Matching

Match each term to its corresponding definition or description. Use each term once.

Definition or Description	**Term**
23. _____ Taken during an acute situation requiring immediate attention	a. Chief complaint
24. _____ Step-by-step evaluation of circumstances	b. Family history
25. _____ History completed the first time a patient is seen	c. Medical history
26. _____ Education, home environment, hobbies	d. Present problem
27. _____ Previous childhood and adult illness	e. Systems review
28. _____ Organized physiologic data	f. Complete history
29. _____ Touches on major points of concern without detail	g. Inventory history
30. _____ Brief description of the perceived problem	h. Focused history
31. _____ A chronicle of events since last meeting with patient	i. Interim history
32. _____ Pedigree diagram	j. Social history

Copyright © 2003, Mosby, Inc. All rights reserved.

Crossword Puzzle

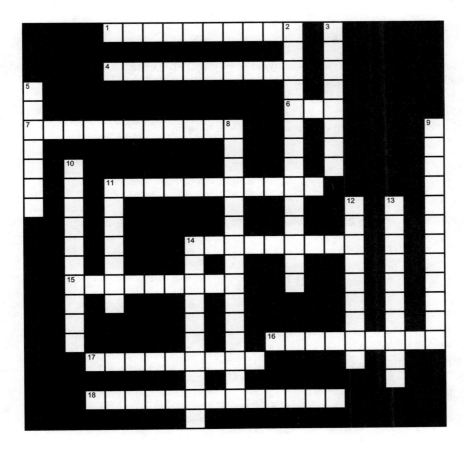

Across

1 Type of treatment modality characterized by inducing a pathologic reaction antagonistic to the condition being treated

4 Repetition of the patient's comments to obtain clarity or confirmation

6 Percentage of patients in population who have other than heterosexual orientation

7 Describes optimal relationship between patient and interviewer

11 Ability of the interviewer to make changes in approach, pace, or focus of the process in order to facilitate obtaining information

14 Words or acronyms used to help remember a series of steps

15 Types of questions that cannot be answered with "yes" or "no"

16 Assessment of variation of intensity or occurrence of a condition

17 Type of history taken if limited time makes a complete history impossible

18 Type of history that reviews milestones achieved by children

Down

2 Types of symptoms including fever, malaise, weight change, or altered sleeping patterns

3 The right of the patient to self-determination

5 Demonstration of acceptance and understanding of the patient

8 A representation of family history of a condition or disease

9 Aspect of the patient's life that encompasses religious and philosophic issues

10 Assessment of patient's ability to complete activities of daily living

11 Type of history taken in case of life-threatening situation

12 Type of history that includes pregnancies and deliveries

13 Type of behavior that characterizes domestic violence

14 Type of history that is important for patients who may be on many prescription and/or nonprescription drugs

Copyright © 2003, Mosby, Inc. All rights reserved.

CONCEPTS APPLICATION

Activity 1

For each of the following scenarios, describe what types of physical examinations would be conducted (complete, focused, problem-oriented, interim). Outline the information you would collect.

1. A mother runs into the emergency room with her 6-year-old son. She says her son fell 15 feet from a tree. You observe a child who is screaming and has an open fracture to the left forearm.

2. A patient presents to a women's health clinic stating she has had a positive home pregnancy test and desires prenatal care.

3. A diabetic comes into the medical clinic stating that he has noticed a sore on his foot for the last week. You note that his last visit was 2 months ago.

Activity 2

Listed in the following table are patient behaviors that can create tension for the examiner. In the blank space provided, indicate a behavior exhibited by the examiner that could help to decrease the tension.

Patient Behavior	Examiner Behavior to Decrease Tension
Seduction	
Dissembling	
Anxiety	
Excessive flattery	
Financial concerns	

Copyright © 2003, Mosby, Inc. All rights reserved.

CASE STUDY

Bill Hogan is a 32-year-old male who presents to the clinic with a complaint of back pain. He tells you he first noticed the pain 2 days ago when he woke up from sleep. Mr. Hogan indicates the pain is a problem because he has been unable to work and it has made him very irritable. He states, "The pain seems to be in the lower back area. It is worse in the morning and late at night, but it comes and goes during the day."

Consider the information you already have, as well as additional information you need to acquire. Using relevant questions—"Where?" "When?" "What?" "How?" and "Why?"—complete the following table. Fill in data you already have in the appropriate areas; then write additional questions to include for each area.

Relevant Question	*Patient Data You Already Know and Questions You Should Ask*
Where?	Data already known: Additional question(s):
When?	Data already known: Additional question(s):
What?	Data already known: Additional question(s):
How?	Data already known: Additional question(s):
Why?	Data already known: Additional question(s):

Copyright © 2003, Mosby, Inc. All rights reserved.

Cultural Awareness

LEARNING OBJECTIVES

After studying Chapter 2 in the textbook and completing this section of the workbook, students should be able to:

1. Define *cultural competence*.
2. Distinguish between ethnic and physical characteristics.
3. Discuss the impact of culture on health beliefs and practices.
4. Describe the cultural impact of disease.
5. Identify questions that explore a patient's culture.
6. Compare and contrast value orientations among cultural groups.

TEXTBOOK REVIEW

Chapter 2   Cultural Awareness (pages 38–48)

CONTENT REVIEW QUESTIONS

Multiple Choice

Circle the correct answer for each of the following questions.

1. Developing cultural sensitivity is vital for the examiner in order to be successful in:
   a. performing a physical examination.
   b. recognizing and accepting beliefs about health that differ from his or her own.
   c. identifying patients at high risk for various diseases.
   d. applying statistical trends of various ethnic and cultural groups.

Copyright © 2003, Mosby, Inc. All rights reserved.

2. The balance of "hot" and "cold" and its relationship to wellness is a concept that:
   a. has been proven to be without validity.
   b. is only characteristic of underdeveloped nations.
   c. has led to poor sanitization practice in many areas of the world.
   d. is held in belief by cultures such as Arab, Chinese, Filipino, and Hispanic.

3. Developing a knowledge base about cultural groups allows the practitioner to:
   a. predict with complete accuracy the behavior and attitude of the patient.
   b. utilize stereotypic judgments to anticipate the patient's need for instruction and support.
   c. understand the behaviors, practices, and problems observed.
   d. change the behavior and/or practices of the patient to conform to health care practice.

4. Which of the following is an example of a cultural characteristic?
   a. skin color
   b. intelligence
   c. skull size
   d. shared belief

5. An integral part of the overall effort to adequately respond to a person in need is:
   a. cultural awareness.
   b. ethnocentric bias.
   c. political correctness.
   d. racial alertness.

6. A young mother brings her infant to the emergency room with a high fever and dehydration. Which of the following questions asked by an examiner demonstrates cultural awareness?
   a. "When did the symptoms begin?"
   b. "What do you think is causing this illness?"
   c. "Has your child been exposed to any sick children recently?"
   d. "What have you already done at home to manage your child's illness?"

7. Which group is most likely to be subjected to invasive cardiac procedures in the United States?
   a. middle-class African-Americans
   b. white males
   c. upper-class females
   d. lower-class Asians

8. A common mistake made by health care professionals is to:
   a. acknowledge the practice of folk or herbal remedies.
   b. adapt health care concepts to meet the needs of individuals of other cultures.
   c. stereotype individuals based on color or ethnic group.
   d. carefully assess the understanding and beliefs of culturally diverse individuals.

9. All of the following are cultural considerations that affect health care except:
   a. eye color, temperature, and visual acuity.
   b. social class, age, and gender.
   c. ethnic traditions, level of education, and family relationships.
   d. religious beliefs, dietary habits, and mode of communication.

10. Which of the following is an example of a physical, as opposed to a cultural, characteristic?
    a. language
    b. hair style
    c. skin color
    d. religious affiliation

Copyright © 2003, Mosby, Inc. All rights reserved.

11. Despite repeated instruction over a period of 3 years, the mother of three young children has still not had them immunized. Which of the following questions would help the health care provider understand this situation?
    a. "When are you going to get your children immunized?"
    b. "What are your beliefs about immunizations?"
    c. "We have asked you to get your children immunized. Why has this not been done?"
    d. "Don't you understand that your children may get ill without immunizations?"

12. Which of the following beliefs is characteristic of a present-oriented individual?
    a. Understands the connection among past events and behaviors and future outcomes.
    b. Anticipates a brighter future; values change as a coping style.
    c. Maintains behaviors that were meaningful in the past; worships ancestors.
    d. Accepts each day as it comes; sees the future as unpredictable.

13. Which modes of communication may be offensive to a patient with different cultural perspective than the practitioner?
    a. Speaking in modulated tones.
    b. Allowing quiet time for reflection during an interview.
    c. Using reflection to repeat the information to obtain clarification.
    d. Maintaining firm and direct eye contact.

14. Which of the following statements are an accurate interpretation of the balance of "hot" and "cold"?
    a. Treatment to restore "hot" and "cold" balance requires the use of opposites.
    b. The recommended treatment for a "cold" condition is to serve "cold" foods.
    c. The recommended treatment for a "hot" condition is "hot" foods and "cold" medications.
    d. Ailments and treatments considered as "hot" or "cold" are related to the effect of body temperature.

Terminology Review

Fill in the blanks in the following statements, selecting the appropriate terms from the word choice box. Terms may be used more than once.

Word Choice Box

primacy   *yin* and *yang*   change   Doing Orientation   cultural competency

---

15. The ability to conscientiously understand a patient's attitudes and beliefs is often defined as _____.

16. A focus on accomplishments is most typically seen with _____.

17. Resistance to _____ is at the root of social and economic tragedy.

18. The forces of "hot" and "cold" are called _____ in Asian cultures.

19. The concept of _____ places the individual patient in the center of a series of concentric circles.

Copyright © 2003, Mosby, Inc. All rights reserved.

Matching

Match each term to its corresponding definition. Use each term once.

Definition

20. _____ Belief that one's own culture is superior to others
21. _____ A physical characteristic not based on culture
22. _____ A habitual activity passed along by family members
23. _____ The act of shedding one culture and assuming another
24. _____ Formal, religious, or other ceremonial acts
25. _____ Behavior approved by group standards
26. _____ Regulating behavior used in different situations
27. _____ Inflexible generalizations about a group
28. _____ The ideas, customs, and behaviors within a group or subgroup
29. _____ A group different than the majority population

Term

a. Stereotype
b. Ritual
c. Race
d. Ethnocentrism
e. Acculturation
f. Minority
g. Values
h. Norm
i. Rite
j. Custom

Copyright © 2003, Mosby, Inc. All rights reserved.

Crossword Puzzle

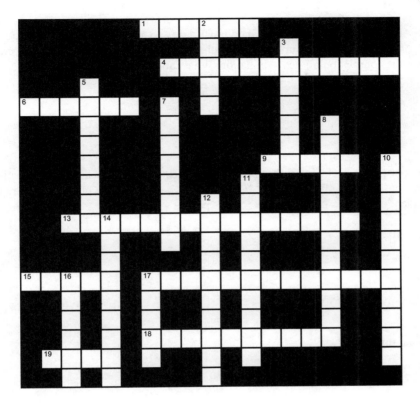

Across

1. The behavioral, cultural, or psychological traits typically associated with one sex
4. Sensitivity or attachment to religious values
6. Legitimate decision-making authority in Asian cultures
9. Orientation that emphasizes self-expression
13. Relational orientation that emphasizes interactions with outsiders
15. Relative worth, utility, or importance
17. Adapting to a culture and taking on its identity
18. A cultural aspect of the socioeconomic profile
19. Orientation that is focused on tradition

Down

2. Orientation that emphasizes accomplishments
3. A group's shared values
5. A "hot" herb that might be used to treat dysmenorrhea
7. View that our lives are a part of a greater whole
8. Typical "hot" condition that might be treated with barley water
10. Decreased diversity within a group
11. Orientation where relationships within one's own level are emphasized
12. Group within a larger culture that has distinctive differentiating traits
14. The phenomenon of various characteristics, values, and behaviors within populations
16. Orientation where group goals dominate over personal goals
17. Group with common culture and distinctive traits

Copyright © 2003, Mosby, Inc. All rights reserved.

CRITICAL THINKING

1. A young Native American child with severe abdominal pain and fever is brought to the clinic by his mother and grandmother. Upon examination, the nurse notes a foul-smelling cloth wrapped around the child's abdomen, which will interfere with the completion of the examination. What should the examiner do?

2. You have a "minority patient" who has a chronic illness requiring dietary teaching and education about medications. Listed below are areas for cultural assessment. For each area, list at least one question that might be asked as part of a cultural assessment in order to better prepare for this patient's care.

    Health beliefs and practices:

    Religious and ritual influences:

    Dietary practices:

    Family relationships and relational orientation:

Copyright © 2003, Mosby, Inc. All rights reserved.

Examination Techniques and Equipment

LEARNING OBJECTIVES

After studying Chapter 3 in the textbook and completing this section of the workbook, students should be able to:

1. Apply standard precautions for infection control to the examination process.
2. Correctly obtain baseline data (vital signs, height, and weight) and describe the meaning of the findings.
3. Identify various types of equipment used for physical examination.
4. Describe the purpose of various types of equipment used for physical examination.
5. Demonstrate the correct use of various types of equipment used for physical examination.
6. Identify various techniques applied during a physical examination.
7. Describe the purpose of various techniques used during a physical examination.
8. Demonstrate correct application of the various techniques used during physical examination.

TEXTBOOK REVIEW

Chapter 3   Examination Techniques and Equipment (pages 49–81)

CONTENT REVIEW QUESTIONS

Multiple Choice

Circle the correct answer for each of the following questions.

1. Which of the following infection control guidelines is currently recommended by the Centers for Disease Control and Prevention (CDC)?
   a. universal precautions
   b. body substance isolation
   c. standard precautions
   d. illness-based precautions

2. A patient presents with multiple raised lesions on her skin. Which instrument should be used to examine these lesions?
    a. calipers
    b. ruler
    c. tympanometer
    d. transilluminator

3. In an outpatient setting such as a clinic, how should infection control practice differ from that in the acute-care setting?
    a. The use of transmission-based precautions is not applicable in an outpatient setting.
    b. Infection control is limited to protecting the outpatient health care provider.
    c. The spread of infection to other patients is not a concern in the outpatient setting.
    d. Infection control practice is applicable in all health care settings.

4. How does an examiner determine the correct size of a blood pressure cuff on an adult? The cuff should:
    a. be 2 1/2 to 3 times the length of the arm.
    b. be able to wrap around the arm once.
    c. cover 25% of the upper arm.
    d. be 40% of the circumference of the arm.

5. How is a blood pressure reading affected if an adult cuff is used on a small child?
    a. Blood pressure readings will be lower.
    b. Blood pressure readings will be higher.
    c. Results will demonstrate a false high systolic reading and a false low diastolic reading.
    d. Blood pressure readings are not affected; cuff size is merely a matter of comfort.

6. The examiner notices an obvious odor to the patient when they first meet. Which examination technique is being applied?
    a. inspection
    b. palpation
    c. percussion
    d. auscultation

7. Focused visual attention obtains data from:
    a. inspection.
    b. palpation.
    c. percussion.
    d. auscultation.

8. Which technique is applied throughout the entire examination and interview process?
    a. inspection
    b. palpation
    c. percussion
    d. auscultation

9. As a component of palpation, which surface is most sensitive to vibration?
    a. fingertips
    b. heel of the hand
    c. dorsal surface of the hand
    d. ulnar surface of the hand

Copyright © 2003, Mosby, Inc. All rights reserved.

10. How deep do the hands press while performing deep palpation?
    a. 1 cm
    b. 2 cm
    c. 4 cm
    d. 8 cm

11. Intensity, related to percussion tones, refers to:
    a. how loud the tone is.
    b. the location of the tone.
    c. the musical quality of the tone.
    d. the length of duration the tone is heard.

12. Indirect finger percussion involves striking the middle finger of the nondominant hand with:
    a. the fist.
    b. a percussion hammer.
    c. the tip of the middle finger of the dominant hand.
    d. a stethoscope.

13. A patient has a urinary tract infection. The examiner wishes to assess tenderness over the kidney. Which examination technique is appropriate?
    a. light finger palpation over the kidney
    b. firm fist percussion over the kidney
    c. deep abdominal palpation of the kidney
    d. auscultation for kidney bruit

14. The examiner has detected a superficial mass in the skin. What part of the hand is best to use to palpate this?
    a. fingertips
    b. heel of the hand
    c. dorsal surface of the hand
    d. ulnar surface of the hand

15. Ideally, auscultation should be carried out last, *except* when examining the:
    a. lungs.
    b. heart.
    c. abdomen.
    d. kidney.

16. Which of the following techniques is *incorrect* and affects the accuracy of auscultation?
    a. placing the stethoscope firmly on the surface to be auscultated
    b. auscultating through clothing
    c. isolating one sound at a time during auscultation
    d. listening for sound characteristics

17. When measuring the length of an infant, the measurement should extend from:
    a. forehead to feet.
    b. crown to tip of toes in prone position.
    c. head to toes in upright position.
    d. crown to heel in supine position.

18. The tubing of a stethoscope should be less than 18 inches long to prevent:
    a. transmission of external noise.
    b. tangling of the tubing in the examiner's clothing or pockets.
    c. distortion of sounds during auscultation.
    d. magnification of the transmitted sounds.

Copyright © 2003, Mosby, Inc. All rights reserved.

19. Which of the following is true regarding correct use of a stethoscope? The:
    a. bell is pressed lightly against the skin to detect low-frequency sounds.
    b. bell is pressed firmly against the skin to hear low-frequency sounds.
    c. diaphragm is pressed firmly against the skin to hear low-frequency sounds.
    d. diaphragm is pressed lightly against the skin to hear high-frequency sounds.

20. The examiner must be sure that the earpieces of the stethoscope are placed so that the alignment fits the contour of the ear canal. In which direction should they be placed? Pointing:
    a. upward
    b. downward
    c. forward
    d. backward

21. In which of the following situations is use of a Doppler indicated?
    a. measurement of body temperature in a hypothermic patient
    b. auscultation of the abdomen in a patient with hypoactive or absent bowel sounds
    c. measurement of blood pressure in a patient with hypertension
    d. auscultation of a nonpalpable pulse in a patient with peripheral vascular disease

22. The red numbers on a lens selector dial of an ophthalmoscope indicate:
    a. that a large amount of light will enter the eye being examined.
    b. that a small amount of light will enter the eye being examined.
    c. positive magnification.
    d. negative magnification.

23. While performing an internal eye examination, the examiner observes a fundal lesion. What feature on the ophthalmoscope permits the examiner to estimate the size and location of the lesion?
    a. grid light
    b. slit light
    c. red-free filter
    d. small light

24. An ophthalmoscope has positive and negative magnification in order to:
    a. compensate for myopia or hyperopia in the examiner's or the patient's eyes.
    b. allow for magnification of both the anterior eye and the posterior eye.
    c. compensate for the degree of dilation of the patient's eyes.
    d. allow for visualization of the eye in patients with normal vision, as well as those with glaucoma.

25. In which of the following situations is the pneumatic attachment of an otoscope indicated?
    a. removal of excessive ear wax from an adult or child
    b. inflation of the ear canal in an adult with a collapsed canal for improved viewing
    c. assessment of pressure behind the tympanic membrane of a child
    d. evaluation of the cone of light reflex in an adult or child

26. The difference between a tuning fork for auditory screening and one for vibratory sensation is the:
    a. sound frequency generated.
    b. strike force placed by the examiner on the forks.
    c. length of the tuning forks.
    d. auditory screening fork is electric; the vibratory fork is not.

27. Very young children may feel threatened by the use of a reflex hammer during examination. What could the examiner use in place of a reflex hammer that would be less threatening?
    a. tuning fork
    b. tongue blade
    c. end of stethoscope
    d. examiner's finger

Copyright © 2003, Mosby, Inc. All rights reserved.

28. According to the Centers for Disease Control, the health care provider should apply infection control measures to which group of patients?
    a. patients with a known infectious disease
    b. patients with a possible infectious disease
    c. patients who appear ill
    d. all patients regardless of their infectious status

29. In which of the following situations is transillumination an appropriate examination technique?
    a. assessment of vesicles on the skin
    b. detection of fluid within the sinuses
    c. measurement of bone density in the skull
    d. determination of a mass in the abdomen

30. Which of the following instruments is used in conjunction with a simple nasal speculum to visualize the lower and middle turbinates of the nose?
    a. otoscope
    b. penlight
    c. ophthalmoscope
    d. goniometer

Terminology Review

Matching

Match each term to its corresponding description or function. Use each term once.

Description or Function	**Term**
31. _____ Used to assess sensation to the plantar surface of the foot	a. Strabismoscope
32. _____ Used to determine the degree of flexion or extension of a joint	b. Aperture setting
33. _____ Instrument with a brush and sharp needle in the base and head	c. Tympanometer
34. _____ Speculum with a bottom blade slightly longer than the top blade	d. Bell of stethoscope
35. _____ Differentiates tissue, fluid, and air within a body cavity	e. Diaphragm of stethoscope
36. _____ Instrument that uses a one-way mirror to detect subtle eye movements	f. Doppler
37. _____ Used to test visual acuity for non-English–speaking patients	g. Goniometer
38. _____ Used to assess function of inner ear	h. Graves' speculum
39. _____ Detects high-pitched sounds	i. Axillary infrared thermometer
40. _____ Used to screen patients at risk for macular degeneration	j. Amsler grid
41. _____ Amplifies sounds by use of ultrasonic waves	k. Episcope
42. _____ Used to inspect the surface of pigmented skin lesions	l. Pederson speculum
43. _____ Used to test visual acuity for literate English-speaking patients	m. Neurologic hammer
44. _____ Adjusts or changes light variations of ophthalmoscope for examination	n. Monofilament
45. _____ Device that correlates with core body temperature of newborn	o. Snellen chart
46. _____ Black light used to detect fungal infections or corneal abrasion	p. "E" chart
47. _____ Detects low-frequency sounds	q. Transilluminator
48. _____ Used for women with small vaginal openings	r. Wood's lamp

Copyright © 2003, Mosby, Inc. All rights reserved.

Crossword Puzzle

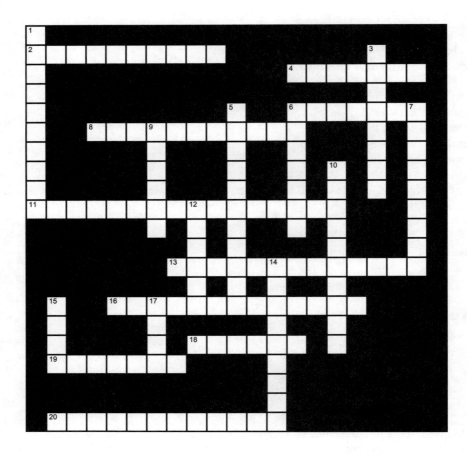

Across

2. Gathering information through sight and smell
4. Type of ultrasonic stethoscope
6. Magnification power of a lens
8. Often a critical diagnostic indicator in infection
11. Instrument used to measure blood pressure
13. Peripheral measurement of cardiovascular function
16. Condition that may be triggered by tactile contact or reaction to cold exam table or stirrups
18. Pulse most often used to assess heart rate
19. Loudest of percussion tones
20. Gathering information through sound

Down

1. Baseline indicators of health status
3. Type of scale used to weigh infants
5. Instrument used to auscultate
6. Determines the degree of percussion tone
7. Sound waves heard as percussion tones
9. Used as a hammer to produce sounds in percussion
10. Gathering information through production of vibrations
12. Grid used to assess for macular degeneration
14. Gathering information through touch
15. Used to percuss internal organs to elicit tenderness
17. The "fifth vital sign"

Copyright © 2003, Mosby, Inc. All rights reserved.

CONCEPTS APPLICATION

Activity 1

List three times when hand washing is indicated in association with an examination.

1.

2.

3.

Activity 2

Complete the following table by providing the expected examination findings.

Area Percussed	Percussion Tone Expected
a. Stomach	
b. Sternum	
c. Lung of patient with emphysema	
d. Liver	
e. Lung of patient with pneumonia	
f. Lung of normal patient	
g. Abdomen with large tumor	

Copyright © 2003, Mosby, Inc. All rights reserved.

CRITICAL THINKING

1. Mrs. Johnson is a 72-year-old female brought to the clinic by her daughter. She has an abdominal fistula draining foul, purulent fluid. She also has bowel and urinary incontinence. What infection control measures should be implemented for Mrs. Johnson?

2. Explain (a) when a nonantimicrobial soap can be used and (b) when an antimicrobial soap is indicated to wash one's hands.

3. Charles Helms comes to the diabetic clinic. He has not been to the clinic in a very long time and tells you he has some problems with his feet. "They just don't feel right," he says.
   a. What type of questions are appropriate to ask Mr. Helms regarding this symptom?

   b. Based on the patient's statement, "They just don't feel right," what are the areas of concern, and how can this be assessed during an examination?

Copyright © 2003, Mosby, Inc. All rights reserved.

4

Mental Status

LEARNING OBJECTIVES

After studying Chapter 4 in the textbook and completing this section of the workbook, students should be able to:

1. Identify aspects of an interview that facilitate mental status examination.
2. Describe techniques to assess mental status in the following areas: physical appearance, cognitive abilities, emotional stability, speech, and language skills.
3. Recognize findings that deviate from expected findings.
4. Compare and contrast common conditions affecting mental status.
5. Identify conditions affecting mental status in various age groups.

TEXTBOOK REVIEW

Chapter 4   Mental Status (pages 82–101)

CONTENT REVIEW QUESTIONS

Multiple Choice

Circle the correct answer for each of the following questions.

1. A patient's inability to follow simple instructions could indicate which of the following findings?
   a. dysphonia
   b. amnesia
   c. aphasia
   d. depression

2. While examining a 14-month-old baby, the examiner observes drooling from the mouth. This finding is:
   a. considered normal.
   b. consistent with mental retardation.
   c. a possible indication of hyperactivity.
   d. commonly associated with cocaine withdrawal.

Copyright © 2003, Mosby, Inc. All rights reserved.

3. A patient scores a 22 out of 40 on a "Set Test" to evaluate mental function as a whole. What does this score indicate?
   a. possible depression
   b. possible dementia
   c. need for further evaluation
   d. normal functioning

4. The examiner asks the patient to complete this statement: "A bird is to air as a fish is to _____." This is an example of what type of testing?
   a. calculation
   b. analogy
   c. judgment
   d. mood and feelings

5. The patient's response to the examiner in question 4 is "scales." What does this response likely reflect?
   a. left cerebral hemisphere lesion
   b. depression
   c. eating disorder
   d. aphasia

6. What technique should be used to evaluate the mental status of a patient with head trauma?
   a. Mini-Mental State
   b. perceptual distortion assessment
   c. Glasgow Coma Scale
   d. functional assessment

7. A patient is nonresponsive and demonstrates a rigid extension of arms, legs, and feet. What does this describe?
   a. decorticate posture
   b. decerebrate posture
   c. hemiplegia
   d. Korsakoff's syndrome

8. Which of the following indicates possible cognitive impairment?
   a. ability to complete personal care without assistance
   b. suspiciousness or inappropriate affect
   c. articulate communication
   d. prudent behavior and calm demeanor

9. A 65-year-old female is brought to the clinic by her family, who report that they have noticed a change in her mental abilities over the past 2 weeks. Normally she is independent, intelligent, and very socially oriented. Her medical history is unremarkable except for congestive heart failure, for which she takes digoxin. She has had no major changes in her health. What question would be the most important for the examiner to ask the family?
   a. "Is there a family history of Alzheimer's?"
   b. "How much alcohol does she drink in an average week?"
   c. "When was her digoxin blood level last checked?"
   d. "Did you know that mental function begins to decline after the age of 60?"

10. A patient who has difficulty writing or drawing is most likely to have which condition?
    a. cerebral dysfunction
    b. peripheral neuropathy
    c. organic brain syndrome
    d. psychiatric hallucinations

Copyright © 2003, Mosby, Inc. All rights reserved.

11. Mrs. Sanders had a cerebrovascular accident 2 days ago. She moves when her name is called. She moans when she experiences painful stimuli. Which of he following best describes Mrs. Sanders' level of consciousness?
    a. confusion
    b. delirium
    c. lethargy
    d. stupor

12. A mother brings her 18-month-old boy to the clinic. She states that the child rarely talks or smiles. She has also noticed he does not like to be held. She states his motor development seems to be normal. These symptoms consistent with what condition?
    a. dementia
    b. autistic disorder
    c. attention deficit
    d. delirium

13. A patient with Alzheimer's will classically display which of the following?
    a. alternating level of orientation—good during the day, but poor at night
    b. hallucinations and decorticate posturing
    c. disintegration of personality
    d. rapid onset of symptoms

Terminology Review

Matching

Match the infant behavior to the age at which you would expect to see it. You will not use every age range.

Infant Behavior	**Age**
14. _____ Babbling, cooing	a. 2 to 3 months
15. _____ Saying,"mama, dada"	b. 3 to 4 months
16. _____ Social smiling	c. 4 to 6 months
	d. 6 to 8 months
	e. 9 to 10 months

Match the information gained to the corresponding area of mental assessment. Answers may be used more than once.

Finding of Examination	**Area of Assessment**
17. _____ Signs of anxiety	a. Cognitive abilities
18. _____ Body language	b. Speech/language
19. _____ Attention span	c. Emotional stability
20. _____ Inability to recall and use words	d. Appearance and behavior
21. _____ Inability to speak in a normal pitch	
22. _____ Alterations in affect	
23. _____ Arithmetic skills	

Copyright © 2003, Mosby, Inc. All rights reserved.

Crossword Puzzle

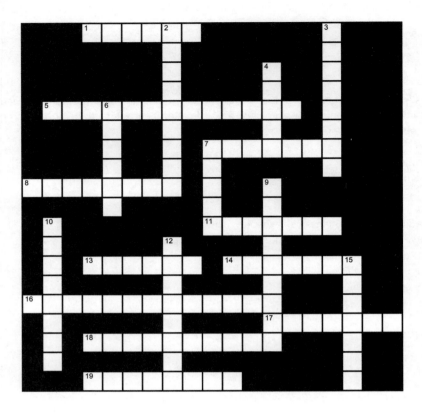

Across

1. Emotional feeling tone
5. Sensory experience not due to external stimulus
7. Inability to complete a task, other than because of paralysis or lack of comprehension
8. Area of temporal lobe that permits comprehension of spoken and written language
11. Coma scale used to assess function of cerebral cortex and brainstem, and to quantify consciousness
13. Part of the cerebrum responsible for perception and behavior
14. Disturbance in ability to express thoughts verbally
16. Demonstrated by patient's ability to follow simple instructions
17. Events in the brain such as trauma, infection, or chemical imbalance
18. Speech defect associated with motor deficit of lips, tongue, palate, or pharynx
19. Ability to reason

Down

2. Impairment of this type is characterized by loss of memory, confusion, inappropriate affect
3. Lobe of the brain primarily responsible for processing sensory data as it is received
4. Area associated with speech formation
6. System that mediates patterns of behavior such as mating, survival, aggression, fear, and affection
7. Associated with decline in synthesis and metabolism of neurotransmitters
9. Disorder of voice volume, quality, or pitch
10. Lobe of brain responsible for perception and interpretation of sounds
12. Lobe of brain primarily responsible for mental status
15. Figure of speech where objects or concepts are compared to each other

Copyright © 2003, Mosby, Inc. All rights reserved.

CONCEPTS APPLICATION

List ways that the following aspects of cognitive abilities might be assessed during examination and how to evaluate the responses.

1. Attention

2. Memory

3. Judgment

4. Insight

5. Abstract reasoning

6. Thought processes and content

Copyright © 2003, Mosby, Inc. All rights reserved.

CASE STUDY

Mrs. Mildred Cobb is a 78-year-old female who is brought to the geriatric clinic by her son and daughter-in-law. Mrs. Cobb's son tells the examiner that his father passed away 5 months ago, and ever since then his mother has "gone downhill." Mr. Cobb indicates that his mother is no longer keeping her house clean or cooking appropriate meals. Also, her personal hygiene habits have changed dramatically. She has lost interest in getting her hair done, and she no longer likes to get dressed for the day. Mr. Cobb tells the examiner, "When I suggest a retirement home, she becomes very angry and tells me to mind my own business. I am just worried about Mom, and I want to make sure she is well cared for." During this conversation, Mrs. Cobb sits quietly. She interjects only to say, "I have taken care of you, your brother, and your father. Now, all of a sudden, you think I am helpless and want to lock me away." Mrs. Cobb appears clean, although her hair is matted and her clothes are badly wrinkled and do not match. Her speech is clear, but her overall affect is very dull. She does not make eye contact with her son or the examiner. A physical examination demonstrates normal bodily functioning consistent with her age group.

1. Which data deviate from normal findings, suggesting altered mental health?

2. What additional questions could the examiner ask to clarify symptoms?

3. What additional physical examination, if any, should the examiner complete?

4. With which conditions affecting mental health are her symptoms consistent?

CRITICAL THINKING

1. What are the types of dementia, and how can they be differentiated?

2. What types of changes in mental functioning can be expected in an older adult? Address personality, intellectual function, problem-solving skills, and memory.

Copyright © 2003, Mosby, Inc. All rights reserved.

Growth and Measurement

LEARNING OBJECTIVES

After studying Chapter 5 in the textbook and completing this section of the workbook, students should be able to:

1. Recognize anatomic and physiologic factors that influence growth.
2. Identify interview methods to gather data pertinent to growth and development.
3. Describe tools and instruments used to assess developmental achievement.
4. Identify expected findings relevant to growth and development throughout the life span.
5. Describe variations in findings that may be considered within normal range.

TEXTBOOK REVIEW

Chapter 5   Growth and Measurement (pages 102–132)

CONTENT REVIEW QUESTIONS

Multiple Choice

Circle the correct answer for each of the following questions.

1. A patient's frame size can be estimated by:
   a. dividing the height by the weight.
   b. dividing height by one-half of the weight.
   c. measuring the head circumference.
   d. measuring the elbow breadth.

2. A 38-year-old female is 5 feet 7 inches tall, weighs 163 pounds, and has a wrist circumference ratio of 11.2 cm. Based on these measurements, the examiner estimates her frame size as:
   a. extra-small.
   b. small.
   c. medium.
   d. large.

Copyright © 2003, Mosby, Inc. All rights reserved.

3. Into what percentile of weight would the patient in question 2 fall? (Refer to Table 5-4 on page 107 in the textbook.)
   a. 45th percentile
   b. 60th percentile
   c. 85th percentile
   d. 90th percentile

4. Eighty percent of brain growth is completed by age:
   a. 1 year.
   b. 2 years.
   c. 4 years.
   d. 7 years.

5. Which cultural group tends to have the highest maturity score of term infants at birth?
   a. African-American
   b. Native American
   c. Caucasian American
   d. Asian American

6. A waist-to-hip circumference ratio over 0.9 in men and 0.8 in women indicates which of the following?
   a. a healthy nutritional status
   b. a low percentage of body fat
   c. a large body frame
   d. an increased risk for disease

7. A child has an arm span that measures greater than his height. With what condition is this finding consistent?
   a. Turner's syndrome
   b. Marfan's syndrome
   c. acromegaly
   d. failure to thrive

8. Growth at puberty is dependent on the interaction of which of the following?
   a. IGF I and sex steroids
   b. FSH and LH
   c. GHRH and IGF I
   d. estrogen and testosterone

9. In the child who fails to thrive, an accompanying lack of emotional attention results in what type of physiologic response?
   a. inability to digest and metabolize nutrients
   b. lack of growth hormone production
   c. excessive thyroid hormone production
   d. neuromuscular degeneration

10. In order to accurately assess height velocity, a child's height must be measured at:
    a. 6-month intervals.
    b. about 9-month intervals.
    c. 12-month intervals.
    d. 14-month intervals.

11. A pregnant patient has a prepregnancy weight-to-height body mass index of 22.4. The examiner expects this patient's weight gain during pregnancy to fall into which weight range?
    a. less than 20 pounds
    b. 20 to 26 pounds
    c. 25 to 35 pounds
    d. 40 to 50 pounds

Copyright © 2003, Mosby, Inc. All rights reserved.

12. Which group of children is typically the heaviest for weight-to-height measurement?
    a. Hispanics
    b. Native Americans
    c. Caucasians
    d. African-Americans

13. The beginning of adolescence is marked by the:
    a. 12th birthday.
    b. development of selfish, impatient behavioral traits.
    c. development of a conscience and a sense of morality.
    d. onset of puberty.

14. To assess and monitor growth, the examiner makes routine measurements of an infant's weight, height/length, and which of the following?
    a. head circumference
    b. hip-to-toe length
    c. forearm length
    d. chest circumference

15. A 4-month-old infant is brought to the clinic. At birth the baby weighed 6 pounds 8 ounces. If the baby is gaining weight at a desired rate, the examiner should expect the baby to now weigh:
    a. 8 pounds.
    b. 9.5 pounds.
    c. 12 pounds.
    d. 15 pounds.

Terminology Review

Word Choice llox
adult stature   gestational age   head circumference   infant stature   SMR (Sexual Maturity Rating)
recumbent length   Ballard Gestational Age Assessment   BMI (Body Mass Index)

Fill in the blanks in the following statements, selecting the appropriate terms from the word choice box Use each term once.

16. The examiner should measure the _____ of a baby with each visit until the age of 2 years.

17. The _____ is a rating to determine a child's pubertal development.

18. The _____ is used to provide guidance in weight gain during pregnancy.

19. A normal finding for _____ is that the patient's sitting height is approximately half the standing height.

20. The _____ is a tool using physical and neuromuscular findings to confirm the gestational age of a newborn.

21. Until 2 or 3 years of age, the baby's height is measured by assessing _____.

22. _____ is an indicator of a newborn's maturity.

23. A normal finding for _____ is that the sitting height is greater than half the standing height.

Copyright © 2003, Mosby, Inc. All rights reserved.

Matching

Match each condition to its corresponding common findings.

	Findings		**Condition**

24. _____ Child with pronounced head enlargement and increased intracranial pressure

25. _____ 5-year-old girl demonstrates pubertal changes

26. _____ 60-year-old man with exaggerated facial features and massive hands

27. _____ 16-year-old female exhibits absence of sexual development; also has short stature and increased carrying angle of elbow

28. _____ Child with normal-sized head and trunk; short, curved arms and legs; dorsal kyphosis and lumbar lordosis

29. _____ Woman with hyperpigmentation to skin, round face, and fat accumulation in lower posterior cervical area

Condition

a. Acromegaly
b. Achondroplasia
c. Cushing's syndrome
d. Hydrocephalus
e. Precocious puberty
f. Turner's syndrome

Crossword Puzzle

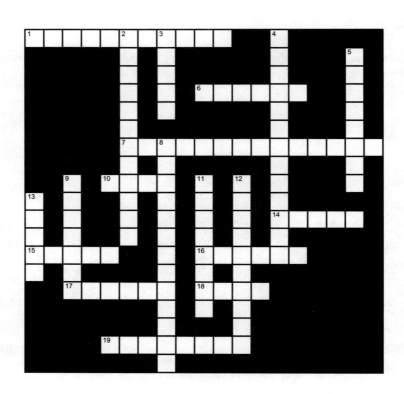

Across

1. Half of individual's ideal weight gained during this period
6. Syndrome of phenotypic females with abnormal sex chromosomes
7. Genetic disorder resulting in abnormalities of endochondrial ossification
10. Growth of this body part predominates during fetal period
14. Growth of this body part predominates during infancy
15. Fetal weight gain peaks during this trimester
16. Gender that develops a wider pelvic outlet during adolescence
17. Increase in size of individual or organ
18. Fastest growing body part during childhood
19. Gestational age is an indicator of this in the newborn

Down

2. Half of body fat present in these tissue layers
3. Body frame size estimated by measuring width of this body part
4. Gestational age used to evaluate this progress
5. Changes in height over a time interval are used to calculate this parameter of growth
8. Result of excessive accumulation of cerebrospinal fluid in the brain or ventricular system
9. Syndrome resulting from chronic excessive cortisol production or long-term administration of glucocorticoids
11. Nutritional status evaluated by measuring thickness of this body part
12. Growth disorder associated with pituitary tumor
13. Age at which stature usually begins to decline

Copyright © 2003, Mosby, Inc. All rights reserved.

CONCEPTS APPLICATION

Baby Michael is a 1-day-old neonate. You have just completed an examination of Michael. Here are the findings you observed:

Measurements

Birth weight: 2300 g   Length: 44.5 cm   Head circumference: 33.0 cm

Neuromuscular Maturity Rating

Posture: 2 points   Square window: 2 points   Ankle dorsiflexion: 2 points
Arm recoil: 1 point   Leg recoil: 1 point   Popliteal angle: 2 points
Heel to ear: 3 points   Scarf sign: 2 points   Head lag: 1 point
Ventral suspension: 2 points

Appearance

Skin: Pale pink with a few large blood vessels noted over the abdomen. Skin has slight thickening with some peeling on the hands and feet. No edema noted.
Lanugo: Some areas of lanugo and bald patches on back of head.
Plantar creases: Slight creases observed over entire heel.
Breast: 2-cm areola diameter, slightly raised. Breast tissue noted on both sides about 0.75 cm.
Ear: Partial incurving of the upper pinna; firm, with instant recoil.
Genitals: Testes descended with moderate rugae.

1. Circle the appropriate boxes on the Newborn Maturity Rating and Classification Form on pages 34 and 35, and determine baby Michael's maturity rating and gestational age based on these findings.

   Maturity rating score = _____   Gestational age = _____

2. Plot baby Michael's measurements for length, weight, and head circumference, using the graphs on page 36.

   Baby Michael's length percentile _____   Baby Michael's weight percentile _____

   Baby Michael's head circumference percentile _____

3. What does the data tell you about baby Michael's gestation and percentile?

Copyright © 2003, Mosby, Inc. All rights reserved.

External sign	Score				
	0	1	2	3	4
Edema	Obvious edema of hands and feet; pitting over tibia	No obvious edema of hands and feet; pitting over tibia	No edema		
Skin texture	Very thin, gelatinous	Thin and smooth	Smooth, medium thickness. Rash or superficial peeling	Slight thickening. Superficial cracking and peeling, especially of hands and feet	Thick and parchmentlike; superficial or deep cracking
Skin color	Dark red	Uniformly pink	Pale pink; variable over body	Pale; only pink over ears, lips, palms, or soles	
Skin opacity (trunk)	Numerous veins and venules clearly seen, especially over abdomen	Veins and tributaries seen	A few large vessels clearly seen over abdomen	A few large vessels seen indistinctly over abdomen	No blood vessels seen
Lanugo (over back)	No lanugo	Abundant; long and thick over whole back	Hair thinning especially over lower back	Small amount of lanugo and bald areas	At least 1/2 of back devoid of lanugo
Plantar creases	No skin creases	Faint red marks over anterior half of sole	Definite red marks over > anterior 1/2; indentations over < anterior 1/3	Indentations over > anterior 1/3	Definite deep indentations over > anterior 1/3
Nipple formation	Nipple barely visible; no areola	Nipple well defined; areola smooth and flat, diameter < 0.75 cm	Areola stippled, edge not raised, diameter < 0.75 cm	Areola stippled, edge raised, diameter > 0.75 cm	
Breast size	No breast tissue palpable	Breast tissue on one or both sides, < 0.5 cm diameter	Breast tissue both sides; one or both 0.5-1 cm	Breast tissue both sides; one or both > 1 cm	
Ear form	Pinna flat and shapeless, little or no incurving of edge	Incurving of part of edge of pinna	Partial incurving whole of upper pinna	Well-defined incurving whole of upper pinna	
Ear firmness	Pinna soft, easily folded, no recoil	Pinna soft, easily folded, slow recoil	Cartilage to edge of pinna, but soft in places, ready recoil	Pinna firm, cartilage to edge; instant recoil	
Genitals Male	Neither testis in scrotum	At least one testis high in scrotum	At least one testis right down		
Female (with hips 1/2 abducted)	Labia majora widely separated, labia minora protruding	Labia majora almost cover labia minora	Labia majora completely cover labia minora		

Copyright © 2003, Mosby, Inc. All rights reserved.

Neurologic signs	Score					
	0	1	2	3	4	5
Posture						
Square window	90°	60°	45°	30°	0°	
Ankle dorsiflexion	90°	75°	45°	20°	0°	
Arm recoil	180°	90°-180°	<90°			
Leg recoil	180°	90°-180°	<90°			
Popliteal angle	180°	160°	130°	110°	90°	<90°
Heel to ear						
Scarf sign						
Head lag						
Ventral suspension						

Total score	Weeks of gestation
0-9	26
10-12	27
13-16	28
17-20	29
21-24	30
25-27	31
28-31	32
32-35	33
36-39	34
40-43	35
44-46	36
47-50	37
51-54	38
55-58	39
59-62	40
63-65	41
66-69	42

Copyright © 2003, Mosby, Inc. All rights reserved.

CLASSIFICATION OF NEWBORNS —
BASED ON MATURITY AND INTRAUTERINE GROWTH
Symbols: X - 1st Exam   O - 2nd Exam

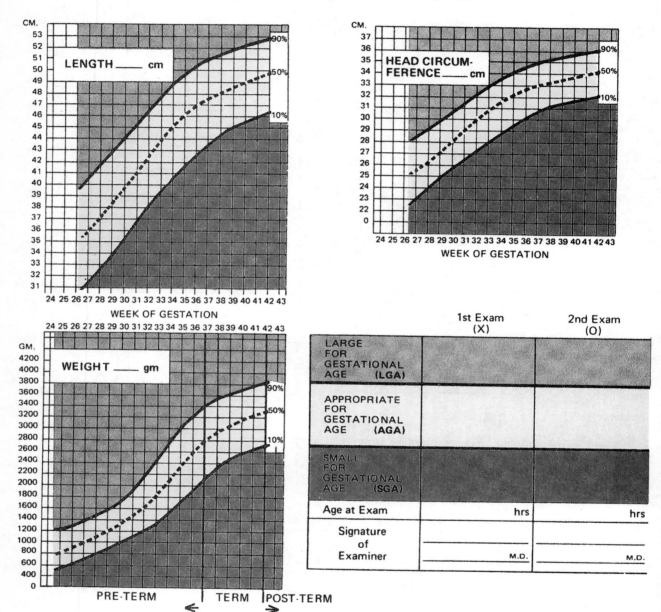

Copyright © 2003, Mosby, Inc. All rights reserved.

6

Nutrition

LEARNING OBJECTIVES

After studying Chapter 6 in the textbook and completing this section of the workbook, students should be able to:

1. Describe interview techniques used to obtain a nutritional history.
2. Identify components of a nutritional examination.
3. Analyze data gained from a nutritional examination.
4. Identify common nutritional conditions.
5. List micronutrients and micronutrients required by the body.

TEXTBOOK REVIEW

Chapter 6   Nutrition (pages 133–162)

CONTENT REVIEW QUESTIONS

Multiple Choice

Circle the correct answer for each of the following questions.

1. During an interview, the patient reports that she frequently has sores at the corners of her mouth. What type of nutritional deficiency should be considered?
   a. vitamin E
   b. protein
   c. B vitamins
   d. fatty acid

Copyright © 2003, Mosby, Inc. All rights reserved.

2. A patient has hypertension but does not have coronary heart disease. If he were to have an LDL level drawn, a diagnosis of hyperlipidemia should be made only if his LDL level is above:
   a. 100.
   b. 120.
   c. 130.
   d. 160.

3. A dietary assessment is performed by:
   a. comparing established eating habits with the recommended dietary allowances.
   b. asking the patient to fill out a food pyramid.
   c. comparing the recommended dietary allowances to the USDA food pyramid.
   d. asking the patient to do a 24-hour dietary recall.

4. Ideally, for an adult, the percentage of total calories coming from fat should be limited to:
   a. 10%.
   b. 30%.
   c. 40%.
   d. 50%.

5. Which of the following laboratory tests is an indicator for protein status of a patient?
   a. albumin
   b. BUN and creatinine
   c. electrolytes
   d. complete blood count

6. A patient has hair that is very dull and easily plucked. The patient is also very thin and appears to have significant muscle wasting. Based on these findings, what other objective data might the examiner anticipate?
   a. thyroid enlargement
   b. hepatomegaly
   c. spongy bleeding gums
   d. ecchymoses and petechiae

7. Healthy eating guidelines recommend _____ servings of the milk, yogurt, and cheese group each day for an adult male.
   a. 1
   b. 2
   c. 3
   d. 5

8. The food guide pyramid recommends 6 to 11 servings from the bread, cereal, and grain products group. Which of the following represents one serving from that group?
   a. 1 cup cooked rice
   b. 6 soda crackers
   c. 1 hamburger bun
   d. 1 slice of bread

9. It is difficult to calculate the exact energy expenditure for a given activity for a specific patient because of individual variables such as:
   a. height.
   b. type of fat cells.
   c. muscle mass.
   d. dietary intake.

Copyright © 2003, Mosby, Inc. All rights reserved.

10. A mother is concerned that her 16-year-old son is not eating enough protein. The young man is 5 feet 5 inches tall and weighs 125 pounds. Referring to Table 6-1, page 134 in the textbook, what is the recommended amount of protein intake?
    a. 45 grams/day
    b. 51 grams/day
    c. 110 grams/day
    d. 112 grams/day

11. Which condition is associated with an increased risk of breast cancer?
    a. exogenous obesity
    b. endogenous obesity
    c. anorexia nervosa
    d. pernicious anemia

12. Physical findings associated with protein deficiency include muscle wasting, dull hair, and:
    a. magenta tongue.
    b. follicular hyperkeratosis.
    c. edema to the extremities.
    d. Bitot's spots.

13. Females from which of the following groups are at the highest risk for eating disorders?
    a. honor-roll students who excel in math and English
    b. teenagers who enjoy eating pizza with friends on the weekend
    c. children from low-income families
    d. college-age students who are perfectionists

14. Which of the following lab values rules out the likelihood that a patient has a vitamin B_{12} deficiency?
    a. serum iron 42 mcg/dL
    b. transferrin saturation 30%
    c. hemoglobin level 14 g/dL
    d. hematocrit level 35%

15. During an examination, a patient tells the examiner she would like to lose weight. She is 5 feet 7 inches tall and weighs 186 pounds. Using a quick estimate for energy needs, how many kcal/kg is appropriate for weight loss for this patient?
    a. 20 kcal/kg
    b. 25 kcal/kg
    c. 30 kcal/kg
    d. 35 kcal/kg

16. The target kcal/day for the patient in question 15 is:
    a. 1642 kcal/day.
    b. 1994 kcal/day.
    c. 2112 kcal/day.
    d. 2412 kcal/day.

17. It is known that the metabolic rate increases after eating. How much of an increase occurs in the total energy expenditure of the body?
    a. 5%
    b. 7%
    c. 10%
    d. 12%

Copyright © 2003, Mosby, Inc. All rights reserved.

18. In order to assess an elderly patient's ability to consume foods, the examiner should:
    a. examine the back, arms, and shoulders for evidence of muscle wasting.
    b. examine the skin for dryness or elasticity.
    c. assess the abdomen for fullness, distension, and bowel sounds.
    d. assess the oral cavity for the condition of the teeth and presence of lesions.

Terminology Review

Fill in the blanks in the following statements, selecting the appropriate terms from the word choice box. Use each term once.

Word Choice Box

exogenous obesity   anthropometrics   bulexaremia   body mass index   cheilosis   Bitot's spots

resting energy expenditure   endogenous obesity   anorexia   midarm muscle circumference

---

19. _____ is a method used to evaluate weight-to-height ratio by dividing the patient's weight by the height in meters squared.

20. The largest proportion of total energy expenditure by the body occurs as a result of _____.

21. The _____ is a sensitive index of protein reserves.

22. A person who has a loss of appetite suffers from _____.

23. _____ is a term that means binge eating followed by self-induced vomiting, usually to control weight.

24. _____ is characterized by an increase in the number of fat cells.

25. _____ are grayish-yellow or white foamy areas seen on the sclera of the eye as a result of vitamin A deficiency.

26. A clinical finding caused by vitamin B_6 deficiency and manifested by reddened lips and fissures at the angles of the mouth is known as _____.

27. _____ is a group of nutritional assessment methods that includes weight for height measurement, body mass index (BMI), skin fold measurement, and midarm circumference.

28. _____ is a condition in which an enlargement of fat cells occurs.

Copyright © 2003, Mosby, Inc. All rights reserved.

Crossword Puzzle

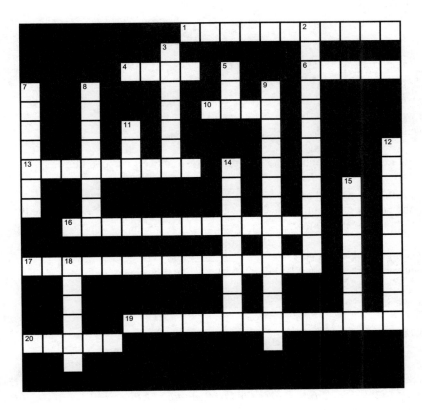

Across

1. Substance associated with coronary heart disease
4. Number of calories in one gram of carbohydrates
6. Number of essential amino acids
10. Nonnutritive eating
13. Type of amino acids that cannot be synthesized in the body
16. Body's main source of energy
17. Procedures for measuring height, weight, skinfold
19. Required and stored by the body in small amounts
20. The most vital nutrient

Down

2. Metabolic response to food intake
3. Disorder characterized by binge eating
5. Formula used to assess nutritional status and total body fat
7. Nutrient made up of amino acids
8. Disorder characterized by perceptual distortion of body shape
9. Term applied to carbohydrates, fats, and proteins because they are required in large amounts by the body
11. Main source of linoleic acid
12. Type of obesity characterized by hypertrophied fat cells
14. Science of food as it relates to health and performance
15. Stored form of carbohydrates
18. Percentage of adult calories that should come from fat

Copyright © 2003, Mosby, Inc. All rights reserved.

CONCEPTS APPLICATION

Activity 1

Consider the following four patients:
    15-year-old male weighing 110 pounds
    25-year-old female weighing 142 pounds
    32-year-old female weighing 200 pounds
    62-year-old male weighing 168 pounds

1. Which of these patients would you guess has the highest resting energy expenditure?

    _____

2. Calculate the resting energy expenditure based on age and body weight for the four patients. Refer to Table 6-9, page 144 in the textbook for assistance.

    15-year-old male weighing 110 pounds: _____ kcal/day
    25-year-old female weighing 142 pounds: _____ kcal/day
    32-year-old female weighing 200 pounds: _____ kcal/day
    62-year-old male weighing 168 pounds: _____ kcal/day

Activity 2

Jack is a 43-year-old male who complains of a loss of energy, loss of appetite, and weight loss. He states that he used to have a steady weight of 172 pounds but that over the last 9 months he has steadily lost weight. Jack is 5 feet 9 inches and currently weighs 142 pounds. He has a midarm muscle circumference of 255 mm.

1. Calculate Jack's desirable weight based on height and weight.
    Desirable body weight _____
2. Calculate Jack's percent of desirable body weight.
    Percent of desirable body weight _____
3. Calculate Jack's percent of his usual weight.
    Percent of usual body weight _____
4. What percent of weight change has Jack experienced with this illness?
    Percent of weight change _____
5. Calculate Jack's current BMI. (Refer to Box 6-4, page 156 in the textbook.) Compare this with his BMI prior to his weight loss.
    Current BMI _____   Previous BMI _____
6. In what percentile does Jack fall in terms of midarm muscle circumference? _____
7. What conclusions can be made regarding the calculations done on Jack?

Copyright © 2003, Mosby, Inc. All rights reserved.

Activity 3

Using the 24-Hour Record of Food Intake form provided on pages 44-46, compile a list of foods you have eaten in the last 24 hours.

Activity 4

Using the Food-Frequency Assessment form on page 47, complete a "typical day" food-frequency assessment for yourself.

Activity 5

Analyze the data you have gathered and compare the results with the suggested daily servings on the Food Guide Pyramid (page 147 in the textbook). Using the nutrition data analysis form below, does your diet meet your nutritional needs?

Nutrition Data Analysis

For each of the food groups, indicate the estimated number of servings eaten each day. Compare this with the recommended number of servings per day. In the last column, indicate whether the intake is below, above, or meets recommended servings.

Food Group	*Estimated # Servings/Day*	*Recommended # Servings/Day*	*Below (B) Above (A) Meets (M)*
Breads, cereals, grains		6–11 servings	
Fruits		2–4 servings	
Vegetables		3–5 servings	
Meat, poultry, fish		2–3 servings	
Milk, cheese, yogurt		2 servings	
Fats, sweets, oils		sparingly	

Copyright © 2003, Mosby, Inc. All rights reserved.

A One-Day (24-Hour) Record of Food Intake

NAME _____   DATE OF RECORD _____

BREAKFAST   Time Eaten _____

Food/Beverage	Type and/or Method of Preparation (List Ingredients.)	Amount
MILK		
FRUIT fresh, canned, sweetened, etc.		
CEREAL _____ with milk _____ with sugar _____ other	Brand _____	
BREAD _____ margarine/butter _____ mayonnaise _____ other	White _____ Brown _____	
EGGS		
MEAT or OTHER PROTEIN		
BEVERAGE _____ with milk _____ with sugar _____ other		
OTHER FOODS		

Did you eat a mid-morning snack?   Yes _____   No _____   If yes, time? _____
(List foods and beverages eaten.)

_____

_____

Copyright © 2003, Mosby, Inc. All rights reserved.

NOON MEAL   Time Eaten _____

Food/Beverage	Type and/or Method of Preparation (List Ingredients.)	Amount
SOUP		
BREAD _____ margarine/butter _____ mayonnaise _____ other	White _____ Brown _____	
_____ MEAT _____ EGG _____ FISH _____ CHEESE		
VEGETABLES _____ cooked _____ raw _____ topping/seasoning (butter, white sauce, cheese sauce, etc.)		
SALAD _____ dressing (brand, etc.)		
FRUIT fresh, canned, sweetened, etc.		
MILK		
BEVERAGE _____ with milk _____ with sugar _____ other		
DESSERT		
OTHER FOODS		

Did you eat an afternoon snack? Yes _____ No _____ If yes, time? _____
(List foods and beverages eaten.)

_____

_____

Copyright © 2003, Mosby, Inc. All rights reserved.

EVENING MEAL   Time Eaten _____

Food/Beverage	Type and/or Method of Preparation (List Ingredients.)	Amount
MAIN DISH _____ meat _____ cheese _____ poultry _____ other protein _____ pasta _____ rice		
VEGETABLES _____ cooked _____ raw _____ topping/seasoning (butter, white sauce, cheese sauce, etc.)		
SALAD _____ dressing (brand, etc.)		
BREAD _____ margarine/butter _____ mayonnaise _____ other	White _____ Brown _____	
FRUIT fresh, canned, sweetened, etc.		
MILK		
BEVERAGE _____ with milk _____ with sugar _____ other		
DESSERT		
OTHER FOODS		

Did you eat an evening snack?   Yes _____   No _____   If yes, time? _____
(List foods and beverages eaten.)

_____

_____

Adapted from Burke B: The dietary history as a tool in research, *J Am Dietic Assoc* 23:1044–1046, 1947.

Copyright © 2003, Mosby, Inc. All rights reserved.

Food-Frequency Assessment

Circle the types of foods and indicate the number of servings you eat of each on a typical day.

Food Group	Amount or Number of Servings
Breads	
Cereal	
Rice/Pasta	
Fruits (type)	
Vegetables (type)	
Milk	
Yogurt	
Cheese	
Meat	
Poultry	
Fish	
Beans	
Eggs	
Nuts	
Fats	
Sweets	
Alcohol	

Copyright © 2003, Mosby, Inc. All rights reserved.

7

Skin, Hair, and Nails

LEARNING OBJECTIVES

After studying Chapter 7 in the textbook and completing this section of the workbook, students should be able to:

1. Conduct a history related to skin, hair, and nails.
2. Discuss examination techniques for skin, hair, and nails.
3. Identify normal age and condition variations to skin, hair, and nails.
4. Recognize findings that deviate from expected findings.
5. Relate symptoms or clinical findings to common pathologic conditions.

TEXTBOOK REVIEW

Chapter 7   Skin, Hair, and Nails (pages 163–224)

CONTENT REVIEW QUESTIONS

Multiple Choice

Circle the correct answer for each of the following questions.

1. Milia are an expected finding in which age group?
   a. newborns
   b. young children
   c. adolescents
   d. older adults

2. An elderly patient asks the examiner, "Is this spot on my chin a cancer?" Which of the following signs or symptoms indicates a need for further medical investigation?
   a. reddish brown color of the lesion
   b. presence on his chin for 20 years
   c. bleeds easily when it is touched
   d. slightly raised and circumscribed

Copyright © 2003, Mosby, Inc. All rights reserved.

3. A 6-year-old girl has freckles over her nose and cheeks. The examiner will recall that freckles are a type of:
   a. macule.
   b. papule.
   c. nodule.
   d. petechiae.

4. The examiner suspects a dark-skinned individual is hypoxic. To assess for the presence of cyanosis, the examiner should:
   a. inspect the skin for a deeper tone of brown or black.
   b. inspect for an ashen-gray color, especially in the mucous membranes.
   c. palpate the skin for a change in moisture and texture.
   d. palpate the skin for changes in skin texture.

5. Why do some infants develop a yellowish skin tone on the third or fourth day of life?
   a. Increased formation of subcutaneous tissue causes a yellow hue.
   b. Capillaries broken during the birth process turn the skin yellow as bruises heal.
   c. Yellowish color results from increased fat metabolism and heat production.
   d. Red blood cells that hemolyze after birth may cause a yellow skin hue.

6. An adolescent patient asks the examiner why teens have more problems with acne than children. Which of the following would be an appropriate response?
   a. "Children have better hygiene habits than adolescents because of parental guidance."
   b. "Adolescents have reduced blood flow to the epidermal layer of the skin, making them more prone to infections."
   c. "At puberty, adolescents begin to secrete more oil from sebaceous glands."
   d. "Children have very little skin mass, which prevents development of acne."

7. Chloasma is an expected finding in which of the following?
   a. newborns
   b. adolescents
   c. pregnant women
   d. older adults

8. While examining the skin of an 87-year-old woman, the examiner observes significant tenting. Which of the following age-associated changes best explains that finding?
   a. Small skin tags form on the neck and back.
   b. The skin becomes thin and takes on a parchment-like appearance.
   c. The skin becomes dry with significant flaking.
   d. There is loss of adipose tissue and loss of elasticity.

9. When assessing for the presence of clubbing, the examiner specifically examines the:
   a. width of the nail base.
   b. angle of the nail base.
   c. thickness of the nail.
   d. color of the nail.

10. Which type of lesion sometimes grows out of an already-present nevus?
    a. malignant melanoma
    b. squamous cell carcinoma
    c. basal cell carcinoma
    d. Kaposi's sarcoma

Copyright © 2003, Mosby, Inc. All rights reserved.

11. In young and school-aged children, the most common skin lesions are due to:
    a. communicable disease and bacterial infection.
    b. changes in skin color and skin tone which accompany puberty.
    c. maturation of melanocytes, which causes changes in skin color.
    d. skin inflammation from sebaceous gland activity.

12. The examiner notes a large blue-black spot on the buttock of a 4-week-old African-American neonate. The mother states that the infant was born with it. The examiner should recognize that this:
    a. is a common finding.
    b. may indicate child abuse.
    c. is related to birth trauma.
    d. suggests a congenital defect.

13. Which of the following may be associated with neurofibromatosis or pulmonary stenosis?
    a. café au lait spots
    b. nevus vasculosus
    c. port wine limb stain
    d. spider angioma

14. Which lesion is an expected finding on the skin of healthy older adults?
    a. acne vulgaris
    b. cherry angioma
    c. miliaria
    d. trichotillomania

15. When palpating skin surfaces for temperature, the examiner should use the:
    a. palmar aspect of the hand.
    b. fingertips of the dominant hand.
    c. dorsal aspect of the hands or fingers.
    d. ulnar surface of the hand.

16. Hyperkeratosis is noted on a patient's palms and soles. The examiner recognizes that this:
    a. may be a sign of a systemic disorder.
    b. may be an indication of a congenital heart defect.
    c. is common among individuals with Down syndrome.
    d. is considered a normal finding.

17. A diabetic patient presents to the clinic complaining of an infected foot. Upon removing the patient's sock, the examiner notes an odor that resembles rotting apples. What type of infection is this consistent with?
    a. *Pseudomonas aeruginosa*
    b. peritonitis
    c. aerobic organism
    d. *Clostridium perfringens*

18. Which finding is consistent with a physical abuse injury in a toddler?
    a. burn to the skin with a splash pattern
    b. bruising of the skin over soft tissue
    c. bruising of the skin over a bony prominence
    d. café au lait patches

19. Which of the following techniques helps the examiner determine whether a palpable skin mass is filled with fluid?
    a. using a Wood's lamp
    b. palpating
    c. transilluminating
    e. noting the odor of the lesion

Copyright © 2003, Mosby, Inc. All rights reserved.

20. Which of the following findings suggests a patient has a fungal infection of the nail beds?
    a. The nail bed is wide and thick.
    b. Nail plate has a central depression, causing a spoon appearance.
    c. Superficial white spots are present in the nail plate.
    d. The nail plate is yellow and crumbling.

Terminology Review

Fill in the blanks in the following statements, selecting the appropriate terms from the word choice box. Use each term once.

Word Choice Box

stellate   vesicle   plaque   confluent   keloid   annular   acrocyanosis   erythema   toxicum   alopecia
serpiginous   dermatomal   reticulate   cutis marmorata   morbilliform   generalized   harlequin
ecchymosis   Mongolian spots   petechiae

---

21. Lesions that run together are referred to as _____.

22. A newborn infant with _____ has cyanosis of the hands and feet.

23. A lesion with a net-like or lacy arrangement is documented as _____.

24. The examiner notes that a patient has hair loss. This is documented as _____.

25. While lying on her side, a newborn infant develops a pink color on the dependent lower half of the body, whereas

    the top half is pale. This finding is known as _____ color change.

26. _____ refers to a star-shaped lesion.

27. A newborn infant develops a pink papular rash with vesicles on the back and thorax 36 hours after birth. This is

    known as _____.

28. Lesions that appear widely distributed or in several areas at the same time are considered

    _____ in distribution.

29. Lesions that appear to occur in a wavy line are referred to as _____.

30. A lesion that forms a ring around a clear center of normal skin is referred to as _____.

31. Areas of deep bluish-gray pigmentation on the sacral aspect of a newborn are referred to as

    _____.

Copyright © 2003, Mosby, Inc. All rights reserved.

32. Hypertrophied scar tissue is referred to as _____.

33. _____ refers to maculopapular lesions that become confluent on the face and body.

34. _____ is a contusion or a bruise.

35. A lesion that follows a nerve or segment of the body is referred to as _____.

36. A fluid-filled, elevated, but superficial skin lesion describes a(n) _____.

37. _____ are tiny, flat, purple or red spots on the skin surface, resulting from minute hemorrhages within the dermal layer.

38. A newborn infant may develop _____ when exposed to decreased temperature.

39. A patient with psoriasis will have a type of skin lesion known as _____.

Matching

Match the disease or condition to the corresponding type of lesion commonly found.

Disease or Condition	Type of Lesion
40. _____ Chicken pox	a. Papule
41. _____ Insect bite	b. Macule
42. _____ Impetigo	c. Vesicle
43. _____ Chronic dermatitis	d. Nodule
44. _____ Lipoma	e. Pustule
45. _____ Blister	f. Patch
46. _____ Wart	g. Lichenification
47. _____ Port wine stain	h. Wheal
48. _____ Petechiae	i. Bulla

Copyright © 2003, Mosby, Inc. All rights reserved.

Crossword Puzzle

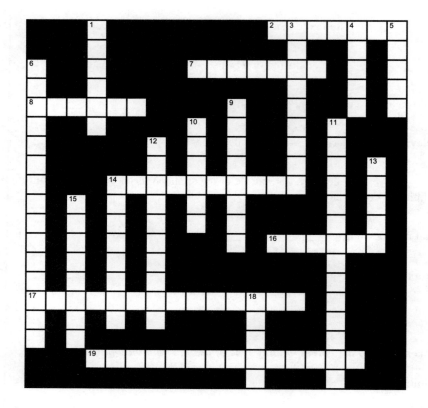

Across

2. Pigment that gives skin its color
7. Waterproofing protein
8. Fine, silky hair of newborns
14. Sweat glands, sebaceous glands, hair, and nails
16. Richly vascular connective tissue layer
17. Fine, irregular, red lines produced by capillary dilation
19. Found in thicker skin on palms and soles

Down

1. Short, fine hair that is nonpigmented
3. Outer portion of skin
4. Epidermal cells converted to hard plates of keratin
5. A mole
6. Where keratin cells are synthesized
9. Mask of pregnancy
10. Mixture of sebum and cornified epidermis
11. Protects body against environmental stressors and water loss
12. Connects dermis to underlying organs
13. Type of lamp used to fluoresce skin lesions
14. Glands found in axillae and anogenital areas
15. Loop of capillaries that supplies nourishment for hair follicles
18. Lipid substance that keeps skin and hair from drying out

Copyright © 2003, Mosby, Inc. All rights reserved.

Anatomy Review

Identify structures on the diagram of the nail by writing the correct term in the corresponding space.

a. _____

b. _____

c. _____

d. _____

e. _____

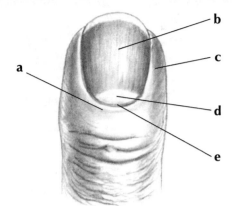

CONCEPTS APPLICATION

Identify the type of secondary lesion in each illustration. Give examples of each type of lesion.

		Name of Lesion	*Examples*
A			
B			
C			
D			

Copyright © 2003, Mosby, Inc. All rights reserved.

CASE STUDY

Mr. John Tate is a 74-year-old male who comes to the clinic for a "routine checkup." Listed below are data collected by the examiner on the patient's skin, hair, and nails.

Interview Data

Mr. Tate denies any specific complaints except that he has some nonpainful sores on his legs that "don't seem to want to heal."

Examination Data

Hair distribution: Full head of hair that is coarse and thinning. No areas of balding noted. Hair color is gray.

Overall appearance of skin: Skin is pale pink, thin, and dry with flaking and tenting present.

Face/Neck: Seborrheic keratoses noted on face. Three cutaneous tags noted on neck. Several senile lentigines noted on neck and face.

Chest/Abdomen: Cherry angiomas noted on chest. Angular surgical scar noted in right upper abdomen.

Extremities: Legs and ankles have areas of erythematous, scaling, and weeping patches. Legs slightly edematous. No hair growth noted on legs. Upper arms: skin very thin and dry; several senile lentigines lesions noted on arms bilaterally.

Nails: Nails are yellowish and thick, but well-trimmed.

1.   What data deviate from normal findings, suggesting a need for further investigation?

2.   What additional questions could be asked by the examiner to clarify symptoms?

3.   What additional examination data should be assessed?

4.   What kind of problem(s) do you think the patient may have?

Copyright © 2003, Mosby, Inc. All rights reserved.

CRITICAL THINKING

1. Mr. Mason is a 72-year-old male who presents to the clinic with a lesion on his cheek. He says it has been there for years, but his wife has been nagging him to "get it checked out in case it is cancer." After examination, you determine the lesion is a benign mole. However, you tell Mr. Mason to "keep an eye on it." What warning signs would you discuss with him?

2. Mrs. Tran brings her 3-year-old child to the pediatric clinic, informing the examiner that the child is "red all over and cries frequently." The examiner notes a rash on the child's skin. What specific characteristics should be noted when examining and documenting a skin lesion?

Copyright © 2003, Mosby, Inc. All rights reserved.

8

Lymphatic System

LEARNING OBJECTIVES

After studying Chapter 8 in the textbook and completing this section of the workbook, students should be able to:

1. Conduct a history related to the lymphatic system.
2. Discuss examination techniques for the lymphatic system.
3. Identify normal age and condition variations to the lymphatic system.
4. Recognize findings that deviate from expected findings.
5. Relate symptoms or clinical findings to common pathologic conditions.

TEXTBOOK REVIEW

Chapter 8   Lymphatic System (pages 225–250)

CONTENT REVIEW QUESTIONS

Multiple Choice

Circle the correct answer for each of the following questions.

1. During an examination, which one of the following questions would be most appropriate for the examiner to ask a patient to elicit information about the lymph system?
   a. "Are you aware of any lumps?"
   b. "Have you had a change in appetite?"
   c. "Do your lymph nodes hurt?"
   d. "Where are your largest lymph nodes?"

2. While palpating lymph nodes on an adult, the examiner should remember that:
   a. tubercular nodes are hot and firm to the touch.
   b. nodes that are fixed and palpable are a normal finding.
   c. heavy pressure is required to locate and identify nodes.
   d. easily palpable nodes are generally not found in healthy adults.

Copyright © 2003, Mosby, Inc. All rights reserved.

3. In comparison with those of a young adult, the lymph nodes on an older adult will be:
   a. large and soft.
   b. small and fatty.
   c. hard and irregular.
   d. large and hard.

4. A 19-year-old male has a severe infection involving the fifth digit of the right hand. Where should the examiner expect to palpate enlarged and tender lymph nodes?
   a. radial aspect of the wrist
   b. palmar aspect of the hand
   c. medial condyle of the humerus
   d. preauricular nodes

5. Which of the following examination findings is cause for concern in an adult?
   a. A palpable lymph node moves under the examiner's fingers.
   b. A palpable lymph node is fixed in its setting.
   c. A palpable lymph node is approximately 3 mm in size.
   d. The lymph node is not palpable.

6. The most common causes of acute suppurative lymphadenitis are which organisms?
   a. *Pseudomonas* and *Clostridium*
   b. *Streptococci* and *Staphylococci*
   c. *Candida* and *Chlamydia*
   d. *Aspergillus* and *Escherichia*

7. The examiner typically will assess the lymph system using which of the following methods? Assess:
   a. the entire lymph system as a unit, exploring all accessible nodes.
   b. both superficial and deep nodes using palpation and a Doppler.
   c. the lymph system region by region as each body system is assessed.
   d. the lymph nodes only when the patient's history suggests a need to do so.

8. A 2-month-old infant is brought to the clinic for immunizations. The examiner palpates enlarged inguinal nodes. What additional finding might explain the enlarged nodes?
   a. The mother reports that the infant suffers from colic.
   b. The infant's length and weight are above the 85th percentile.
   c. The infant has a severe diaper rash.
   d. A port wine stain is present on the infant's left thigh.

9. As the examiner palpates an enlarged lymph node, the patient complains of pain. This is an indication of:
   a. an inflammatory process.
   b. Hodgkin's disease.
   c. immature lymph node development.
   d. malignancy.

10. Which examination method is used to differentiate an enlarged lymph node from a cyst?
    a. palpation
    b. auscultation
    c. biopsy
    d. transillumination

11. Which of the following methods best describes how to assess supraclavicular lymph nodes?
    a. Place the patient in a supine position and ask the patient to hold his or her breath.
    b. Place the patient in the Trendelenburg position, then illuminate the lymph nodes with a bright light.
    c. Palpate deeply behind the clavicles as the patient takes a deep breath.
    d. Palpate lightly below the clavicles with the patient in a sitting position leaning forward.

Copyright © 2003, Mosby, Inc. All rights reserved.

12. The examiner notes enlarged tonsils on a young child. The examiner should recognize that this:
    a. is an indication of a retropharyngeal abscess.
    b. may be an early indication of Epstein-Barr virus.
    c. is an indication that the child has lymphoma.
    d. may be a normal finding.

13. In addition to the head, neck, axillae, and inguinal area, the examiner may also assess lymph nodes in which location?
    a. on the palmar aspect of the hands
    b. in the popliteal region
    c. in the patellar region
    d. on the dorsum of the foot

14. A patient with tuberculosis is most likely to have which finding?
    a. hard and fixed nodes
    b. pulsating lymph nodes
    c. "cold" lymph nodes
    d. lymph node cysts

15. Which of the following is an assessment technique that can differentiate mumps from cervical adenitis?
    a. palpating the angle of the jaw
    b. palpating enlarged lymph nodes
    c. noting painful lymph nodes
    c. noting swelling of the face

Terminology Review

Matching

Match the disease or condition to its corresponding clinical findings.

Disease or Condition	Clinical Finding
16. _____ Acute lymphangitis	a. Characterized by a large, tender, firm node with overlying tissue that is swollen and red
17. _____ Acute suppurative lymphadenitis	b. Manifested in a young child who has fever, is restless and drooling, and sits up and hyperextends his neck to breathe
18. _____ Hodgkin's disease	c. Nonpitting edema to the extremities with thick overlying skin
19. _____ Retropharyngeal abscess	d. Red streaking moving up an extremity accompanied by fever
20. _____ Cat scratch fever	e. Nodal enlargement lasting longer than 3 weeks in a young child
21. _____ Lymphedema	f. Asymmetric enlargement of the cervical lymph nodes, which are rubbery, nonpainful

Copyright © 2003, Mosby, Inc. All rights reserved.

Anatomy Review

On the diagram below, complete the following activities:

1. Draw in the palpable lymph nodes in various regions.

2. Label the various regions of the lymph nodes that you have drawn.

3. Indicate with a number (1–6) the order in which you would palpate the head for lymph node examination.

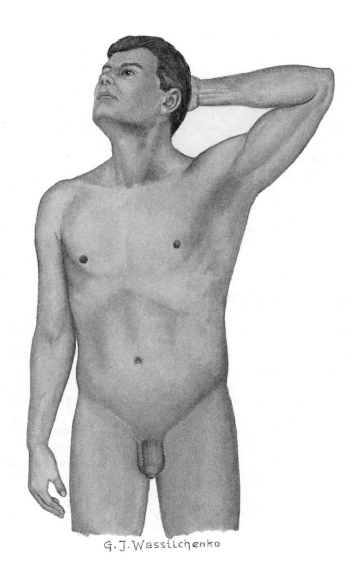

G. J. Wassilchenko

Copyright © 2003, Mosby, Inc. All rights reserved.

CASE STUDY

Mario is a 16-year-old male complaining of fatigue and weakness. Listed below are data collected by the nurse during an interview and examination.

Interview Data

Mario indicates he keeps a busy schedule with school, basketball, and work. He has always been a good student, but he seems to be having a harder time keeping up with everything. He feels he is beginning to let his family and friends down because fatigue and weakness are interfering with his performance at school and on the basketball court. Mario does not want to quit his job because he is saving for college. When asked about other symptoms, he denies changes in appetite or abdominal problems but reports that he thinks he sometimes has a fever.

Examination Data

General survey: Alert, thin male. Height 5 ft 7 in. Weight 140 pounds.

Skin: Skin color is pink. No evidence of bruising. No skin discoloration.

Thorax: Respirations even and unlabored, clear to auscultation. Heart rate and rhythm regular.

Abdomen: Bowel sounds auscultated. Abdomen soft, nontender, and nondistended.

Musculoskeletal: Moves all extremities; symmetrical. Moves joints without tenderness.

Head and neck: Enlarged and firm cervical lymph nodes. Supraclavicular nodes also palpable.

1. What data deviate from normal findings, suggesting a need for further investigation?

2. What additional questions could be asked by the examiner to clarify symptoms?

3. What additional examination data should be assessed?

4. What kind of problem(s) do you think the patient may have?

Copyright © 2003, Mosby, Inc. All rights reserved.

CRITICAL THINKING

1. While examining a young adult female patient, you palpate enlarged lymph nodes. Identify the "nine S's" to consider when examining the lymph nodes.

2. How does the lymph system examination vary from an infant or young child to an adult to an older adult? Indicate how findings change with aging.

Copyright © 2003, Mosby, Inc. All rights reserved.

Head and Neck

LEARNING OBJECTIVES

After studying Chapter 9 in the textbook and completing this section of the workbook, students should be able to:

1. Conduct a history related to the head and neck.
2. Discuss examination techniques for the head and neck.
3. Identify normal age and condition variations to the head and neck.
4. Recognize findings that deviate from expected findings.
5. Relate symptoms or clinical findings to common pathologic conditions.

TEXTBOOK REVIEW

Chapter 9   Head and Neck (pages 251–277)

CONTENT REVIEW QUESTIONS

Multiple Choice

Circle the correct answer for each of the following questions.

1. In which group is a slight enlargement of the thyroid gland considered a normal finding?
   a. infants
   b. adolescents
   c. pregnant women
   d. Native Americans

2. The examiner notes a nodule on the thyroid gland of a 42-year-old male. What additional finding is suggestive that this may be malignant, requiring further evaluation? The:
   a. patient's voice has become progressively hoarse over the last few months.
   b. examiner palpates multiple nodes on both lobes of the thyroid.
   c. cervical lymph nodes are not palpable.
   d. patient states that his mother and sister both have bumps on their thyroids.

Copyright © 2003, Mosby, Inc. All rights reserved.

3. Which of the following questions is appropriate to ask a female patient with a suspected thyroid problem?
   a. "How much alcohol do you drink?"
   b. "Have you noticed a change in your sleep pattern or energy level?"
   c. "Do you have headaches?"
   d. "Are you currently menstruating?"

4. An infant with an alcoholic mother is admitted to the hospital with fetal alcohol syndrome. What assessment finding is consistent with this syndrome?
   a. ear dysplasia
   b. moon face
   c. torticollis
   d. thin upper lip

5. Which of the following findings in an elderly patient would be considered a normal process of aging?
   a. narrowed palpebral fissures
   b. pulsating fontanels
   c. uneven movement of the tongue
   d. fibrosis of the thyroid gland

6. Assessment of an infant's fontanels is best performed while the infant is:
   a. calm and in an upright position.
   b. sleeping in a lateral position.
   c. supine and awake.
   d. held at a 45-degree angle.

7. A patient reports a severe headache accompanied by nausea, vomiting, and intolerance to light. These symptoms are consistent with which type of headache?
   a. temporal
   b. migraine
   c. cluster
   d. traumatic

8. A 6-month-old infant is brought to the clinic for immunizations. While examining the baby, the examiner notes that the anterior fontanel has not closed. What is the significance of this finding? This:
   a. indicates a slight developmental delay.
   b. suggests a nutritional deficiency.
   c. is consistent with hydrocephaly.
   d. is a normal finding.

9. What clinical finding may accompany thyroid hypertrophy in hyperthyroidism?
   a. multiple nodules on thyroid gland
   b. indentation of thyroid gland in the right and left lobes
   c. vascular bruit auscultated over thyroid gland
   d. swelling of the face

10. Preterm infants often have:
    a. long, narrow heads.
    b. broad nose bridges.
    c. low-set ears.
    d. webbed necks.

Copyright © 2003, Mosby, Inc. All rights reserved.

11. The presence of a nodular thyroid is a normal finding in:
    a. infants.
    b. adolescents.
    c. pregnant women
    d. older adults.

12. Neck webbing, excessive posterior cervical skin, and a short neck are signs associated with:
    a. Asian heritage.
    b. chromosomal anomalies.
    c. Cushing's syndrome.
    d. malnutrition.

13. Transillumination of the skull should be performed:
    a. on infants of diabetic mothers.
    b. on infants with a history of traumatic birth.
    c. when an infant has a facial nerve palsy.
    d. on infants with suspected intracranial lesions.

14. Which of the following findings suggests an inflammation of the thyroid gland?
    a. gritty sensation when the thyroid is palpated
    b. movement of the thyroid when patient swallows
    c. vertical ridges palpated on the thyroid gland
    d. swollen and red skin overlying the thyroid gland

15. A patient demonstrates asymmetry of the mouth. The examiner suspects a problem with the:
    a. inferior facial nerve.
    b. thyroid gland.
    c. peripheral trigeminal nerve.
    d. salivary duct.

Terminology Review

Matching

Match each type of headache to its corresponding characteristic.

Type of Headache

16. _____ Hypertensive headache
17. _____ Classic migraine
18. _____ Muscular tension headache
19. _____ Headache from temporal arteries
20. _____ Cluster headache

Characteristic

a. May be brought on by extreme anger
b. May be brought on by alcohol consumption
c. Associated with a well-defined prodromal event
d. Begins in morning and decreases as day progresses
e. Age of onset typically older adult

Copyright © 2003, Mosby, Inc. All rights reserved.

Crossword Puzzle

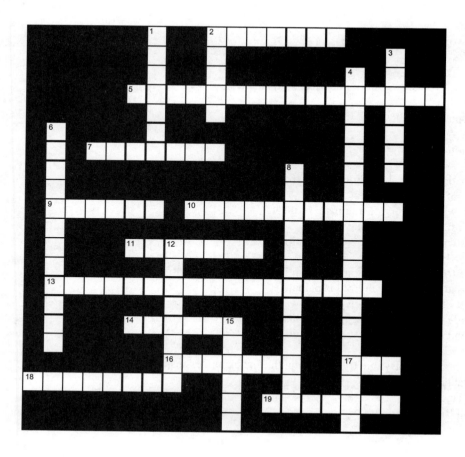

Across

2. Condition of fontanel that may indicate increased intracranial pressure
5. Results from premature closing of sutures
7. Result of shifting and overlapping of bones during vaginal delivery
9. Appearance of face, head, neck that is characteristic of a condition
10. Wry neck
11. Sign associated with increased intracranial pressure after fontanels are closed
13. Procedure to evaluate suspected intracranial lesion or increasing head circumference in infants
14. Thyroid disease characterized by exophthalmia
16. Expected position of trachea
17. Spasmodic contractions of face, head, or neck
18. Characterized by mucinous edema of face
19. Excessive posterior cervical skin

Down

1. Largest endocrine gland
2. May be detected in hypervascular thyroid
3. Third fontanel common in Down syndrome
4. Extends from upper sternum to mastoid process
6. Begins in sutures after brain growth is completed
8. Protrusion of nervous system tissue through a defect in the skull
12. "Mask of pregnancy"
15. Produced by parotid, submandibular, and sublingual glands

Copyright © 2003, Mosby, Inc. All rights reserved.

Anatomy Review

On the diagram below, identify the structures in the neck by writing the correct term in the corresponding lettered answer space. Use each term once.

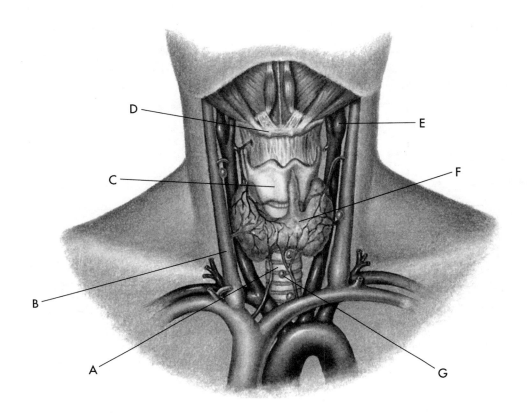

carotid artery   lymph node   cricoid cartilage   thyroid gland

hyoid bone   trachea   jugular vein

a. _____   e. _____

b. _____   f. _____

c. _____   g. _____

d. _____

Copyright © 2003, Mosby, Inc. All rights reserved.

CONCEPTS APPLICATION

Complete the table below by providing the differences in the physical appearance and demeanor of a patient with hyperthyroidism and one with hypothyroidism.

System or Structure	Hyperthyroidism	Hypothyroidism
Weight		
Emotional state		
Temperature preference		
Hair		
Skin		
Neck		
Gastrointestinal		
Eyes		

CASE STUDY

Rob is a 44-year-old carpenter who comes to the emergency room complaining of a severe headache. Listed below are data collected by the examiner.

Interview Data

When the examiner attempts to ask Rob about the headache, he cries out, "I can't take this any more—it hurts too much." His wife says that Rob has been getting these headaches a couple of times a day for the last week now—sometimes at night—so he has not been sleeping well. She also indicates that he had headaches like these about a year ago and that they lasted about a month. When Rob is asked if he experiences nausea or sensitivity to light, he replies, "No, I just get a stuffy nose." His wife says that Rob is constantly worried about whether—and when—the headache will come back because, as she says, "We don't know what is causing them, and nothing seems to help them go away." She says Rob feels like all he can do is hold his head and pray that the pain will stop.

Copyright © 2003, Mosby, Inc. All rights reserved.

Examination Data

General survey: Alert, well-nourished male of average weight, in moderate distress. He is unable to lie still and paces the floor around the examination area, holding the left side of his head (over his eye and forehead).

Head and neck: Skull is intact, with no lumps, depressions, or tenderness. No abnormalities are found with facial structures. The head is centered on the neck; the trachea is midline. Thyroid is in midline position and of normal size.

1. What data deviate from normal findings, suggesting a need for further investigation?

2. What additional questions could be asked by the examiner to clarify symptoms?

3. What additional examination data should be assessed?

4. What kind of problems do you anticipate this patient will have?

Copyright © 2003, Mosby, Inc. All rights reserved.

CRITICAL THINKING

1. What role does the technique of percussion play in the examination of the head and neck?

2. What role does the technique of auscultation play in the examination of the head and neck?

Copyright © 2003, Mosby, Inc. All rights reserved.

10

Eyes

LEARNING OBJECTIVES

After studying Chapter 10 in the textbook and completing this section of the workbook, students should be able to:

1. Conduct a history related to the eyes and vision.
2. Discuss examination techniques for the eyes.
3. Identify normal age and condition variations to the eyes.
4. Recognize findings that deviate from expected findings.
5. Relate symptoms or clinical findings to common pathologic conditions.

TEXTBOOK REVIEW

Chapter 10   Eyes (pages 278–312)

CONTENT REVIEW QUESTIONS

Multiple Choice

Circle the correct answer for each of the following questions.

1. Which of the following is relevant information for a history and examination of a child's eyes and vision?
   a. immunization history
   b. growth milestones
   c. birth weight
   d. academic performance

2. Prior to instilling a mydriatic eye drop, the examiner should:
   a. assess the corneal reflex.
   b. observe the eye with focused light tangentially.
   c. assess intraocular pressure.
   d. observe the eye for vascular changes.

3. Which physiologic change with aging explains why an elderly individual may be unaware of an infection or injury to an eye?
   a. decreased corneal sensitivity
   b. diminished tearing
   c. reduced visual acuity
   d. increased density of the lens

4. The examiner screens a 5-year-old child for nystagmus by:
   a. assessing visual acuity.
   b. inspecting the macula of the eye with an ophthalmoscope.
   c. inspecting movement of the eyes to the six cardinal fields of gaze.
   d. palpating the globe while the child holds eyelids closed.

5. Which of the following correctly describes the method to assess accommodation?
   a. Shine a light into the pupil; note constriction.
   b. Note constriction as gaze shifts from across the room to an object 6 inches away.
   c. Note ocular movement as patient follows an object through the six cardinal fields.
   d. Cover one eye of patient with card, then remove the card; note any deviation from a fixed gaze.

6. While testing visual acuity of an adult using a Snellen chart, the patient is able to read all of the letters on the 20/30 line and three letters of the 20/20 line with the right eye. How is this documented?
   a. O.D. 20/30 +3
   b. O.D. 20/20
   c. O.S. 20/20 -4
   d. O.U. 20/30 -3

7. Which of the following should be used to test for near vision?
   a. Rosenbaum chart
   b. Snellen "E" chart
   c. confrontation test
   d. cover-uncover test

8. In order to visualize the macula, the examiner should ask the patient to:
   a. blink eye several times quickly.
   b. lie in a supine position.
   c. look directly into the light of the ophthalmoscope.
   d. direct eye gaze on an object to the left, and then to the right.

9. Which of the following statements made by a parent should make the examiner suspicious of a visual problem in a baby? "My:
   a. 2-week-old baby seems to see a toy in front of her, but she does not follow it when it moves."
   b. 4-month-old daughter cannot seem to distinguish colors."
   c. 1-month-old baby does not seem to be able to control his eye movements."
   d. 3-month-old son does not seem to see things placed in front of him."

10. A 51-year-old patient tells the examiner, "My mother had glaucoma. What can I do to prevent myself from getting it?" Which of the following responses is most appropriate?
    a. "It is prevented by avoiding chronic eye irritation."
    b. "Limiting the exposure of ultraviolet light to the eye will prevent glaucoma."
    c. "Since it is inherited, you will eventually get it, and there is nothing you can do to stop that."
    d. "Although it can't be prevented, regular screening and testing assists in early detection."

Copyright © 2003, Mosby, Inc. All rights reserved.

11. Until 6 years of age, eyeballs are less spherical than those of adults, which accounts for why children have:
    a. ciliary muscle weakness.
    b. myopic acuity.
    c. lens rigidity.
    d. a lack of red reflex.

12. Which of the following is considered a routine part of a newborn examination?
    a. assessing red reflex
    b. assessing extraocular movements with six fields of gaze
    c. funduscopic examination
    d. visual acuity

13. Which examination finding may be indicative of a retro-orbital tumor?
    a. episcleritis
    b. Argyll Robertson pupil
    c. unilateral exophthalmos
    d. retinitis pigmentosa

14. A patient tells the examiner, " I have a loss of vision in the outer half of each eye." Which of the following underlying problems should the examiner consider?
    a. diabetes
    b. pituitary tumor
    c. glaucoma
    d. cytomegalovirus (CMV) infection

15. Which of the following data is an applicable component to family history?
    a. eye dominance
    b. pupil size
    c. retinoblastoma
    d. sty

16. Mrs. Carter has vision that, at best, is 20/210. Mrs. Carter is considered:
    a. legally blind.
    b. mildly myopic.
    c. moderately hyperopic.
    d. unilaterally anisocoric.

17. Which of the following is the correct technique while performing an ophthalmoscopic examination? Examine the patient's right:
    a. eye with your right eye, and the left eye with your left eye.
    b. eye with your left eye, and the left eye with your right eye.
    c. and left eyes with your dominant eye.
    d. and left eyes with your nondominant eye.

18. Failure to elicit a red-reflex in a young child may indicate:
    a. congenital glaucoma.
    b. myosis.
    c. retinopathy.
    d. retinoblastoma.

19. An examiner is most likely to observe pseudostrabismus in which of the following groups?
    a. older adults
    b. Native American infants
    c. pregnant women
    d. Hispanics

Copyright © 2003, Mosby, Inc. All rights reserved.

20. A cobblestone appearance of the conjunctiva is most likely related to:
    a. subconjunctival hemorrhage.
    b. allergic or infectious conjunctivitis.
    c. lagophthalmos.
    d. cytomegalovirus infection.

Terminology Review

Matching

Match each clinical finding with its corresponding associated factor.

<table>
<tr><td>**Clinical Finding**</td><td>**Associated Factor**</td></tr>
<tr><td>21. _____ Adie pupil</td><td>a. Acute angle glaucoma</td></tr>
<tr><td>22. _____ Anisocoria</td><td>b. Congenital finding in 20% of normal population</td></tr>
<tr><td>23. _____ Argyll Robertson pupil</td><td>c. Diabetic neuropathy or alcoholism</td></tr>
<tr><td>24. _____ Mydriasis</td><td>d. Oculomotor nerve damage</td></tr>
<tr><td>25. _____ Eye deviated laterally, downward</td><td>e. Neurosyphilis or midbrain lesion</td></tr>
<tr><td>26. _____ Durban bodies</td><td>f. Lipid disorder</td></tr>
<tr><td>27. _____ Corneal arcus</td><td>g. Senile macular degeneration</td></tr>
</table>

Copyright © 2003, Mosby, Inc. All rights reserved.

Crossword Puzzle

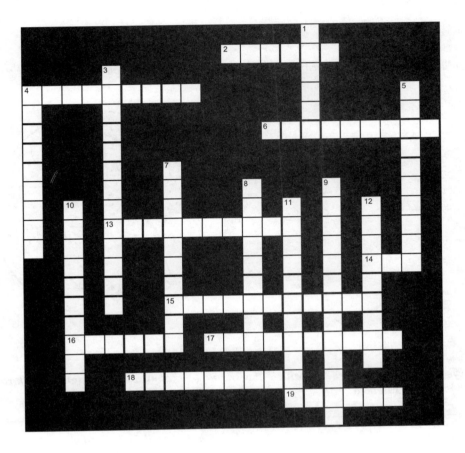

Across

2. Drooping upper eyelid
4. Eyelid turned inward
6. Involuntary dysrhythmic movement of the eyes
13. Inequality of pupillary size
14. Reflex caused by light illuminating retina
15. Loss of definition of the optic disc
16. Also known as fovea
17. Defective vision in half of the visual field
18. Abnormal growth of conjunctiva that extends over the cornea from the limbus
19. Grid used to evaluate central vision

Down

1. Pupillary constriction
3. Test for estimating peripheral vision
4. Lower eyelid is turned away from the eye
5. White spots found on the iris and usually associated with mental retardation
7. Loss of accommodation
8. A sty caused by staphylococcal organisms
9. Eyes widely spaced apart
10. Both eyes do not focus on the same object simultaneously
11. Elevated plaque of cholesterol commonly found on the nasal portion of the lid
12. Pupillary dilation

Copyright © 2003, Mosby, Inc. All rights reserved.

CONCEPTS APPLICATION

Activity 1

Referring to the following illustration, describe the position of the lesion based on disc diameter.

Location _____

Length _____

Width _____

Optic disc

Lesion

Activity 2

List the external eye structures in the order in which they should be examined. To the right of each structure, identify what specifically should be examined.

Structure	What Should Be Examined
1.	
2.	
3.	
4.	
5.	
6.	
7.	

Copyright © 2003, Mosby, Inc. All rights reserved.

CASE STUDY

Andy is a 32-year-old single white male who has insulin-dependent diabetes mellitus. His reason for seeking care is a vision problem. Listed below are data collected during an interview and examination.

Interview Data

Although Andy has been compliant, he has had poor control of his diabetes. He presents to the clinic with complaints of significant reduction in vision over the last couple of weeks. Andy tells the nurse, "I can't lose my vision because I won't be able to keep my job. If I can't see, I don't know how I will take care of my diabetes or how I will maintain my income."

Examination Data

General survey: Anxious, well-nourished male.

Eyes: Snellen test O.S. 20/70, O.D. 20/70 +2, O.U. 20/60 +1; reduced peripheral vision. Normal extraocular movement and corneal light reflex. Eyelids and eyelashes symmetric. Conjunctiva clear bilaterally. Sclera is white; corneas clear. Lacrimal structures without tearing. Pupils are equal and round and react to light.

Internal eye exam: Retinal vessels hemorrhagic. New vessels present. Findings consistent with proliferative diabetic retinopathy.

1. What data deviate from normal findings, suggesting a need for further investigation?

2. What additional questions could the examiner ask to clarify symptoms?

3. What additional examination, if any, should the nurse complete?

4. What problem or problems does this patient have?

Copyright © 2003, Mosby, Inc. All rights reserved.

CRITICAL THINKING

1. A 5-year-old child is brought in for a routine physical examination. Describe what components of eye examination are appropriate for a child of this age without specific eye or visual complaints.

2. While examining the eye, the examiner notes retinal vessels. How are arteries and veins differentiated?

Copyright © 2003, Mosby, Inc. All rights reserved.

Ears, Nose, and Throat

LEARNING OBJECTIVES

After studying Chapter 11 in the textbook and completing this section of the workbook, students should be able to:

1. Conduct a history related to the ears, nose, and throat.
2. Discuss examination techniques for the ears, nose, and throat.
3. Identify normal age and condition variations to the ears, nose, and throat.
4. Recognize findings that deviate from expected findings.
5. Relate symptoms or clinical findings to common pathologic conditions.

TEXTBOOK REVIEW

Chapter 11   Ears, Nose, and Throat (pages 313–355)

CONTENT REVIEW QUESTIONS

Multiple Choice

Circle the correct answer for each of the following questions.

1. When performing a Weber test, which of the following is considered a normal finding? The patient:
   a. hears the tone equally in both ears.
   b. hears the tone better in one ear than in the other.
   c. hears sounds longer when conducted through air than when conducted through bone.
   d. is able to detect tones of varying frequencies and pitches from a tuning fork.

Copyright © 2003, Mosby, Inc. All rights reserved.

2. Which of the following best explains why infants and toddlers are at greater risk for ear infections than are older children and adults?
    a. poorly developed immune system
    b. immature tympanic membrane
    c. wider, shorter, and horizontal eustachian tube
    d. excess deposition of bone cells along the ossicle

3. Which finding is most likely to suggest a foreign object in the nose of a young child? The:
    a. mother states that the child plays with toys.
    b. examiner notes a purulent discharge from the child's nose.
    c. child has a foul-smelling odor from the nose.
    d. child cries when lying down.

4. The examiner observes a blackish lesion on the top surface of the tongue of an adult patient. The patient indicates that his tongue is painful. Which question by the examiner would be helpful in explaining this finding?
    a. "Have you been taking antibiotics lately?"
    b. "Have you injured your tongue?"
    c. "Have you been diagnosed with mouth cancer before?"
    d. "When was the last time you brushed your teeth?"

5. Which of the following situations is an indication for transillumination? The:
    a. patient complains of epistaxis.
    b. patient has crepitus with jaw movement.
    c. parotid gland is palpable and tender.
    d. patient complains of pain over sinuses with palpation.

6. The examiner is examining the ears of a school-aged child who has a tympanostomy tube in the left ear. Which of the following is an expected finding for the tympanic membrane of this ear?
    a. bulging without mobility
    b. retracted with limited mobility
    c. chalky white in appearance
    d. amber-colored appearance

7. The examiner notes that a patient's tonsils are enlarged and touch the uvula. This is documented as:
    a. 1+.
    b. 2+.
    c. 3+.
    d. 4+.

8. A patient complains of dizziness and a "whirling" sensation. Which of the following questions by the examiner would be helpful in explaining this finding?
    a. "When was the last time you went swimming?"
    b. "Are you taking any medications?"
    c. "Have you noticed any discharge coming from your ears?"
    d. "Do you work or live in an environment where there is a lot of noise?"

9. An adult patient with a history of an upper respiratory infection complains of severe vertigo and hearing loss on one side. What examination technique should be used to evaluate equilibrium for suspected vestibular dysfunction?
    a. Weber test
    b. transillumination
    c. Schwabach test
    d. Romberg test

Copyright © 2003, Mosby, Inc. All rights reserved.

10. Which of the following statements made by a parent should raise the examiner's suspicion that the tympanic membrane of a young child has ruptured?
    a. "She has some bloody, yellowish-looking stuff coming out of her ear."
    b. "She has been crying all night, but feels better this morning."
    c. "My child has had a fever and earache."
    d. "My child's earwax is dark brown."

11. Which of the following statements made by a 72-year-old patient would indicate a normal process of aging?
    a. "My tongue feels swollen."
    b. "My tonsils are large and sore."
    c. "Food does not taste the same as it used to."
    d. "I have white and black spots under my tongue."

12. Which of the following behaviors, as described by a parent, may indicate that an infant or young child may have a hearing problem?
    a. "My 4-month-old baby does not seem to respond to loud noises."
    b. "My 5-month-old baby is babbling, but she is not yet saying any words."
    c. "Sometimes my 3-year-old does not pay attention to me."
    d. "When my 15-month-old baby is talking, I sometimes have a hard time understanding her."

13. An infant born weighing less than 1500 grams is at risk for:
    a. otosclerosis.
    b. hearing loss.
    c. cleft lip and palate.
    d. choanal atresia.

14. While examining the ear of a 6-week-old infant, the examiner observes a tympanic membrane lacking conical appearance and with a diffuse light reflex. These findings:
    a. suggest a congenital abnormality.
    b. suggest a ruptured tympanic membrane.
    c. are classic findings for otitis media in the neonate.
    d. are normal.

15. Chronic sniffling, nasal congestion, nosebleeds, mucosal scabs, and septum perforation are signs of:
    a. chronic allergies.
    b. cocaine abuse.
    c. fungal infection.
    d. turbinate hypertrophy.

Copyright © 2003, Mosby, Inc. All rights reserved.

Terminology Review

Fill in the blanks in the following statements, selecting the appropriate terms from the word choice box.

Word Choice Box

Darwin tubercle   Epstein's pearls   Nylen Barany   Koplik's spots   malocclusion

---

16. The examination for vestibular function disorder is the _____ test.

17. White specks with a red base found on the buccal mucosa opposite the first and second molars are known as

    _____ and may occur in a child with a fever or with rubeola.

18. A _____ appears as a blunt point projecting up from the upper part of the helix of the ear.

19. Improper position of the teeth is referred to as _____.

20. On the roof of the mouth of an infant, _____ appear as small whitish masses and are considered a normal finding.

Matching

Match each clinical finding with its corresponding associated factors.

Clinical Finding	Associated Factors
21. _____ Labyrinthitis	a. Dry mouth, systemic disease
22. _____ Meniere's disease	b. Fever, headache, nasal discharge
23. _____ Sinusitis	c. Vertigo, nystagmus
24. _____ Tonsillitis	d. Ear fullness, tinnitus
25. _____ Xerostomia	e. Dysphagia, fever, fetid breath

Copyright © 2003, Mosby, Inc. All rights reserved.

Crossword Puzzle

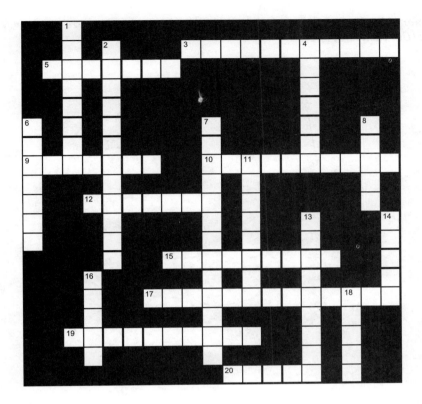

Across

3. Bilateral sensorineural hearing loss associated with aging
5. Dizziness
9. Used to screen for equilibrium
10. Located between the mouth and nasopharynx
12. Spots that appear on buccal mucosa; ectopic sebaceous glands
15. Dry, cracked lips
17. "Swimmer's ear"
19. Dry mouth
20. Bony protuberance on lingual surface of mandible

Down

1. Attaches tongue to floor of mouth
2. Ossification that results in fixation of stapes
4. Coiled structure in inner ear
6. Earwax
7. Epithelial growth migrating through tympanic membrane
8. Projecting shell-like structure on the side of the head; auricle
11. Malleus, incus, and stapes
13. Nosebleed
14. Suspended from the posterior margin of the soft palate
16. Tests lateralization of sound
18. Compares bone conduction with air conduction of sound

Copyright © 2003, Mosby, Inc. All rights reserved.

Anatomy Review

On the illustration below, identify the structures of the middle ear by writing the correct term in the corresponding lettered answer space. Use each term once.

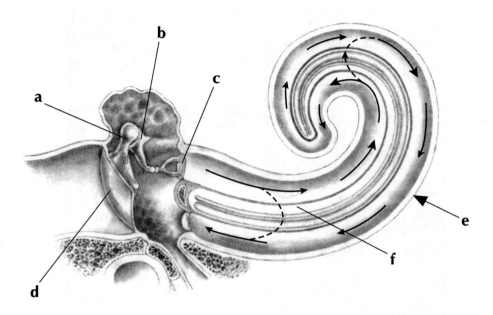

cochlea	malleus
cochlear duct	stapes
incus	tympanic membrane

a. _____

b. _____

c. _____

d. _____

e. _____

f. _____

Copyright © 2003, Mosby, Inc. All rights reserved.

CASE STUDY

Trudy is a 5-year-old Native American girl who was brought to the clinic by her mother. Listed below are data collected by the examiner during an interview and examination.

Interview Data

The mother tells the examiner, "Trudy has been complaining of ear pain. She has been very hot and crying frequently." She adds, "I wanted to bring Trudy to the clinic yesterday, but my grandmother told me I shouldn't." Trudy's mother continues, telling the examiner, "Trudy has been treated many times for this problem over the last several years by the medicine man. Last night I saw drainage from Trudy's ears. Grandmother told me this was a sign that the illness was being chased from the body. I did not know what it was, but I felt scared." The mother indicates that Trudy knows English, but that the girl has never really talked very much.

Examination Data

General survey: Small-for-age 5-year-old girl; quiet, flat affect. Does not look at the examiner; does not interact with the mother or the examiner.

External ear exam: Typical position of ears bilaterally. Left ear pinna red. Dried bloody drainage noted on left external ear and in left external canal. Cries when left ear is touched. Right ear unremarkable.

Internal canal and tympanic membrane: Dried drainage noted in the left ear canal. TM perforated. Right ear unremarkable.

Hearing examination: Whisper test in right ear = 80%; Whisper test in left ear = 0%. Weber test: hears tuning fork in right ear.

1. What data deviate from normal findings, suggesting a need for further investigation?

2. What additional questions could the examiner ask to clarify symptoms?

3. What additional physical examination, if any, should the examiner complete?

4. What primary problems does the patient have?

Copyright © 2003, Mosby, Inc. All rights reserved.

CRITICAL THINKING

1. A mother brings her 6-month-old infant to the clinic and tells the examiner, "She has had a fever all night and has been crying for the last hour." The examiner looks in the baby's ears and notes that the tympanic membrane is red. How can the examiner differentiate redness caused by otitis media from redness caused by crying?

2. What is the primary cause of sleep apnea, and why is it a concern?

Copyright © 2003, Mosby, Inc. All rights reserved.

Chest and Lungs

LEARNING OBJECTIVES

After studying Chapter 12 in the textbook and completing this section of the workbook, students should be able to:

1. Describe anatomy and physiology of the chest and lungs.
2. Describe interview questions pertinent to chest and lung examination.
3. Identify appropriate equipment used for chest and lung examination.
4. Discuss inspection, palpation, percussion, and auscultation techniques for examination of the chest and lungs.
5. Identify age-specific variations in chest and lung examination.
6. Identify examination findings associated with various conditions of the chest and lungs.

TEXTBOOK REVIEW

Chapter 12   Chest and Lungs (pages 356–413)

CONTENT REVIEW QUESTIONS

Multiple Choice

Circle the correct answer for each of the following questions.

1. As the chest of a newborn is examined, bowel sounds are auscultated in the chest. What is the significance of this finding? This is:
   a. a normal finding in newborns.
   b. an abnormal but benign finding in children until age 2.
   c. abnormal and possibly indicates an enlarged liver.
   d. abnormal and possibly indicates a diaphragmatic hernia.

Copyright © 2003, Mosby, Inc. All rights reserved.

2. Which of the following patients demonstrates the highest risk factor for respiratory disability?
   a. a patient with a history of hypertension
   b. a child who has had a previous respiratory infection
   c. a patient with paraplegia
   d. an extremely thin female patient

3. An adult male patient complains of a "persistent cold that will not go away." He is a nonsmoker; his skin color is normal. Which one of the following is most important to this patient's history?
   a. allergy tests and treatment plans
   b. expectations for treatment and care
   c. experiences with difficult breathing
   d. previous sports injuries and rehabilitation

4. The health care professional is examining the chest of a 22-year-old female who is 8 months pregnant. The patient has a wide thoracic cage. Which of the following best explains this finding?
   a. She may have lung disease, such as emphysema.
   b. She may be hypoxic and may require oxygen supplementation.
   c. She may be pregnant with twins, causing abdominal contents to be forced up and out.
   d. This is considered a normal finding with advanced pregnancy.

5. In which of the following conditions should the examiner expect the costal angle to be greater than 90 degrees?
   a. chronic obstructive pulmonary disease
   b. pneumothorax
   c. infant respiratory distress syndrome
   d. atelectasis

6. Which of the following findings indicates respiratory distress in the infant or young child?
   a. respiratory rate of 30 breaths per minute
   b. irregular respiratory pattern
   c. observation of sternal and supraclavicular retractions with breathing
   d. auscultation of bronchovesicular sounds throughout the lung field

7. The examiner notes a diaphragmatic excursion of 4 cm on the right side and 8 cm on the left side. What do these findings mean?
   a. The patient may have a pleural effusion.
   b. The patient may have a pneumothorax.
   c. Asymmetrical findings are common in well-conditioned adults.
   d. This is a normal finding because the right lung is larger than the left lung.

8. During percussion, the patient holds his or her arms in front in order to:
   a. expose maximum lung area.
   b. make the ribs protrude.
   c. prevent attacks of coughing.
   d. reduce discomfort.

9. Which of the following examination techniques is not typically done when examining the chest and lungs of a newborn?
   a. general survey
   b. inspection
   c. percussion
   d. auscultation

Copyright © 2003, Mosby, Inc. All rights reserved.

10. The patient tells the examiner, "I have been coughing up a lot of yellowish-green phlegm." The examiner should suspect:
    a. viral infection.
    b. tuberculosis.
    c. pulmonary edema.
    d. bacterial pneumonia.

11. In order to best visualize subtle retractions on a patient, the examiner should:
    a. place the patient in a supine position.
    b. stand directly behind the patient.
    c. ensure that the light source angles toward the patient.
    d. position the patient directly under a bright examination light.

12. Which of the following findings could indicate an intrathoracic infection?
    a. malodorous breath
    b. protrusion of the clavicle
    c. clubbing of the nail beds
    d. Kussmaul's respirations

13. Which finding is considered unusual for a newborn?
    a. sneezing
    b. coughing
    c. prominence of xiphoid process
    d. nose breathing

14. In the older adult, which finding can occur in the absence of disease as a result of age-related changes of the chest or lungs?
    a. hyperresonance
    b. productive cough
    c. asymmetric expansion of the chest
    d. pulmonary infiltrate

15. A newborn infant with a small chest-to-head size ratio is usually associated with:
    a. maternal diabetes.
    b. cocaine use during pregnancy.
    c. intrauterine growth retardation.
    d. a normal finding.

16. Hamman's sign can best be heard when the patient is:
    a. in a supine position.
    b. lying on the left side.
    c. sitting completely upright.
    d. positioned with the head elevated 30 degrees.

17. In addition to severe respiratory distress, which of the following findings may be indicative of a pneumothorax with mediastinal shift?
    a. hemoptysis
    b. pleural friction fremitus
    c. vesicular lung sounds over the peripheral lung field
    d. tracheal deviation away from midline position

Copyright © 2003, Mosby, Inc. All rights reserved.

18. A mother tells the examiner that her 2-year-old child has a cough that "sounds just like a bark." Given this history, what other findings should the examiner anticipate with respiratory examination?
    a. wheezing and coarse crackles bilaterally
    b. labored breathing and inspiratory stridor
    c. hyperresonance with percussion
    d. productive, blood-tinged, or "rusty" sputum

19. A 4-year-old child is brought to the emergency department. The examiner notes Kussmaul's respirations of 50 per minute. The child has no fever, no cough; good air movement in lungs, with no abnormal breath sounds auscultated. Which of the following questions would be most helpful for the examiner to ask the parents?
    a. "What is his normal respiratory rate?"
    b. "What would you like for me to do for him?"
    c. "Do you think he may have swallowed a toy?"
    d. "Where do you keep your medications at home?"

20. Which type of apnea is considered normal?
    a. deglutition apnea
    b. secondary apnea
    c. sleep apnea
    d. apneustic apnea

21. The best time to evaluate vocal and tactile resonance on a young child is while the child is:
    a. lying down, asleep.
    b. lying down, awake.
    c. sitting quietly in parent's lap.
    d. crying.

22. The examiner should expect that the ratio of respiratory rate to heart rate is approximately:
    a. 1:2.
    b. 1:4.
    c. 1:6.
    d. 1:8.

23. A patient with long-standing COPD has come to the clinic complaining that his breathing is getting more difficult over the last couple of weeks. Which of the following questions would best help the examiner understand the hypoxia a patient is experiencing?
    a. "Do you think oxygen will help you?"
    b. "In what way has your activity level been affected?"
    c. "Do you have a cough?"
    d. "Have you been taking your medications?"

24. A patient has an undiagnosed tumor in the middle lobe of the right lung, which has caused atelectasis. What finding would exist that might make the examiner suspicious of this problem?
    a. low-pitched grating sound heard during inspiration and expiration
    b. hyperresonance in right middle lobe
    c. diminished or absent breath sounds in right middle lobe
    d. coarse crackles auscultated throughout lung field

25. Which examination finding is consistent with emphysema?
    a. decreased tactile fremitus
    b. dullness with chest percussion
    c. trachea in midline position
    d. an ammonia-like odor on the patient's breath

Copyright © 2003, Mosby, Inc. All rights reserved.

Terminology Review

Matching

Match the type of respiration on the left with the correct description on the right.

Type of Respiration

26. _____ Kussmaul's
27. _____ Cheyne-Stokes
28. _____ Biot's
29. _____ Hamman's sign
30. _____ vesicular
31. _____ bronchovesicular
32. _____ crackles
33. _____ rhonchi
34. _____ wheeze
35. _____ vocal resonance
36. _____ bronchophony
37. _____ pectoriloquy
38. _____ egophony

Description

a. Irregular breaths varying in depth and interrupted by intervals of apnea but lacking repetitive pattern; associated with increased intracranial pressure
b. Low-pitched, low-intensity sounds heard over healthy lung tissue
c. Sonorous wheezes
d. Spoken word transmitted through lung fields; usually muffled and indistinct
e. Increase of intensity of spoken sound with accompanying nasal sound
f. Deep and usually rapid; associated with metabolic acidosis
g. Whisper can be clearly heard through the stethoscope; associated with consolidation of lungs
h. Intervals of apnea followed by crescendo/decrescendo sequence of breathing; often associated with dying
i. Typically moderate in intensity; heard over major bronchi
j. Mediastinal crunch; variety of sound including loud crackles and clicking or gurgling sounds; associated with mediastinal emphysema
k. Continuous, high-pitched musical sound; almost a whistle; heard on inspiration or expiration
l. Abnormal sound, more often heard on inspiration; characterized by discrete discontinuous sounds; rales
m. Greater clarity and increased loudness of spoken words

Copyright © 2003, Mosby, Inc. All rights reserved.

Crossword Puzzle

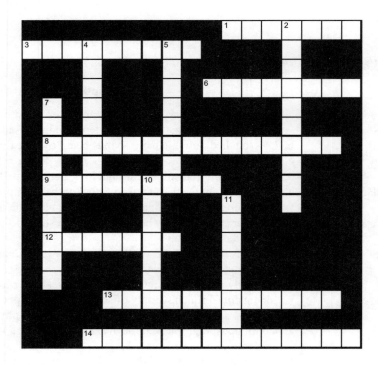

Across

1. Costal angle at the base of this structure where ribs separate
3. Dyspnea while lying down
6. Vibration sensation palpated over the chest while the patient speaks
8. Juncture also known as angle of Louis
9. Dyspnea increases in an upright posture
12. Location of pectus carinatum
13. Caused by accumulation of air in the pleural space
14. Sound commonly percussed over the lung field of a patient with COPD

Down

2. Barrel-chested patient's ribs are more like this
4. Type of breathing one would expect to observe in a patient with an acute rib fracture
5. Accumulation of excess nonpurulent fluid in the pleural space
7. Coughing up blood
10. Serous membranes enclosing the lungs
11. Crinkly sensation palpated on the chest; indicates air in the subcutaneous tissue

Copyright © 2003, Mosby, Inc. All rights reserved.

CONCEPTS APPLICATION

Activity 1

In the table below are pairs of respiratory conditions that may have similar findings. For each pair of conditions, write the examination technique that will allow the examiner to differentiate between the two. Choose from these techniques: percussion, auscultation, tactile fremitus, or sputum analysis. Support your answers.

Conditions	*Similar Findings*	*Examination Technique*
Tuberculosis vs. pneumonia	Dyspnea, fever, malaise, productive cough	
Pneumothorax vs. atelectasis	Dyspnea, diminished breath sounds	
Pneumonia vs. pleural effusion	Fever, shortness of breath, dullness to percussion	
Asthma vs. emphysema	Dyspnea, diminished lung sounds, diminished fremitus	

Activity 2

1. On the illustration below, indicate the location of the lung sounds you should expect to hear with auscultation of the anterior chest, using "B" for bronchial sounds, "BV" for bronchovesicular sounds, and "V" for vesicular sounds.
2. Indicate the location of the manubrium with "M" and the angle of Louis with "AL."
3. Indicate the location of the costal angle with "CA."

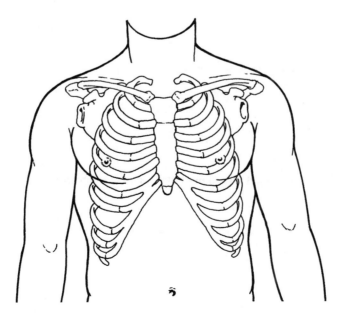

Copyright © 2003, Mosby, Inc. All rights reserved.

CASE STUDY

Sharon is a 66-year-old female complaining of shortness of breath. Listed below are initial data collected during an interview and examination.

Interview Data

Sharon says she's had breathing problems "for years" but is getting worse. She tells the examiner that she gets short of breath with activity, adding that she can do things around the house for only a few minutes before she has to sit down to rest and catch her breath. She says she can sleep only a couple of hours at a time. She sleeps best with two pillows at night, but on some nights she just sits in a chair. Sharon does not currently use oxygen, but she thinks oxygen would help. She admits to smoking 1 1/2 packs of cigarettes a day. She has never quit because she says she just can't do it.

Examination Data

General survey: Alert and slightly anxious female, sitting slightly forward, with moderately labored breathing. Skin is pale with slight cyanosis around the lips and in nail beds. Appears extremely thin.

Chest wall configuration: Chest is round-shaped and symmetrical with increased AP diameter and costal angle greater than 90 degrees. Small muscle mass noted over chest; ribs protrude.

Breathing effort: Respiratory rate 24 and labored.

Chest assessment: Chest wall expansion with respirations is reduced, but symmetrical. Chest wall tactile fremitus diminished. Sibilant rhonchi are auscultated throughout lung field. Lung sounds are diminished in lung bases bilaterally.

Vocal sound auscultation: Muffled tones auscultated.

1.   What data deviate from normal findings, suggesting a need for further investigation?

2.   What additional questions could the examiner ask to clarify symptoms?

3.   What additional physical examination, if any, should the examiner complete?

Copyright © 2003, Mosby, Inc. All rights reserved.

4. What kind of problems do you anticipate this patient will have?

CRITICAL THINKING

1. Mr. Louis Jackson is a 72-year-old male who is seen in the clinic for a routine examination. During the interview Mr. Jackson tells the interviewer that he smokes. When questioned further, he indicates he has been smoking "roughly 60 years." He states, "I started smoking cigarettes when I was about 14 years old. Until I was about 25, I smoked a pack maybe every 3 days or so. Then I started smoking about a 1/2 pack a day until the age of 40. Since that time, I've smoked about a pack a day." Mr. Jackson adds, "I knew I should quit, but I never really wanted to very much. I decided that when I got up to a pack a day, I would never smoke more than that."

    Based on the information given, calculate Mr. Jackson's pack-year history.

2. Mr. Pena is a 41-year-old migrant worker from Mexico who comes to the clinic where you work. Through an interpreter, you learn he has had a fever with night sweats, fatigue, frequent coughing with reddish sputum and weight loss. What significance do these symptoms have?

3. Mrs. Marino tells you all three of her children have had problems with coughing and some trouble breathing ever since they moved into a new apartment 2 months ago. She also tells you they have not had fevers with these symptoms. What type of interview questions should be asked to further explore these symptoms?

Copyright © 2003, Mosby, Inc. All rights reserved.

13

Heart

LEARNING OBJECTIVES

After studying Chapter 13 in the textbook and completing this section of the workbook, students should be able to:

1. Describe anatomy and physiology of the heart.
2. Identify age and condition variations in the heart.
3. Describe interview questions pertinent to the heart examination.
4. Discuss inspection, palpation, percussion, and auscultation techniques for examination of the heart.
5. Describe age-specific and/or condition-specific variations in examination findings of the heart.
6. Identify examination findings associated with various conditions of the heart.

TEXTBOOK REVIEW

Chapter 13   Heart (pages 414–461)

CONTENT REVIEW QUESTIONS

Multiple Choice

Circle the correct answer for each of the following questions.

1. Dextrocardia is a condition characterized by which of the following? The:
   a. right side of the heart is enlarged.
   b. heart is to the right of the stomach.
   c. heart is positioned to the right, either rotated or displaced.
   d. blood sugar in the heart is higher than in other organs.

2. While auscultating the heart of an obese patient, the examiner should expect the heart sounds to be:
   a. louder and closer.
   b. softer and more distant.
   c. louder and more distant.
   d. softer and closer.

Copyright © 2003, Mosby, Inc. All rights reserved.

3. The examiner is unable to palpate the apical pulse. In addition, the heart sounds are very faint to auscultation. What condition should be considered?
    a. pleural or pericardial fluid
    b. congestive heart failure
    c. mitral valve regurgitation
    d. atrial septal defect

4. What disease process should the examiner consider if a patient reports a several-week history of fever and shows clinical symptoms of congestive heart failure?
    a. bacterial endocarditis
    b. infarction
    c. myocarditis
    d. cardiac tamponade

5. In order to accommodate the increased maternal blood volume in the pregnant woman, the:
    a. heart rate drops in order to deal with greater cardiac output.
    b. plasma volume decreases in order to allow for more erythrocytes.
    c. left ventricle increases in both wall thickness and mass.
    d. heart is shifted in position towards a more vertical orientation.

6. The examiner suspects a patient has pulmonary hypertension. What examination findings are consistent with this?
    a. decreased intensity of S_1 heart sounds; increased intensity of S_2 heart sounds
    b. a thrill palpated in area of apex
    c. paradoxic splitting of S_1 and S_2 heart sounds
    d. pericardial friction rub

7. Which of the following cardiac changes occur at birth in the normal child?
    a. the foramen ovale opens
    b. pressure in the right atrium rises
    c. the ductus arteriosus closes
    d. the relative mass of the left ventricle decreases

8. In most adults the apical impulse should be visible at the:
    a. midaxillary line in the fifth right intercostal space.
    b. sternal notch.
    c. midclavicular line in the fifth left intercostal space.
    d. costovertebral angle.

9. While palpating the precordium, a heave is identified, with lateral displacement of the apical pulse. Such a finding may indicate:
    a. mitral regurgitation.
    b. aortic stenosis.
    c. left ventricular enlargement.
    d. pericarditis.

10. A thrill generally indicates which of the following?
    a. a disturbance in the electrical conductivity of the heart
    b. a disruption of blood flow related to defect of closure in the semilunar valves
    c. the presence of massive infection of the myocardium
    d. pulmonary hypotension

Copyright © 2003, Mosby, Inc. All rights reserved.

11. Since percussion has a limited value in determining heart size, left ventricular size is better judged by:
     a. auscultation of the heart sounds.
     b. location of the apical pulse or PMI.
     c. palpating the left sternal border.
     d. palpating the heart base.

12. Which of the following is easily mistaken for cardiac-generated sounds?
     a. bowel sounds
     b. pulmonary insufficiency
     c. pericardial friction rub
     d. tracheal shifting

13. Cardiac tamponade is:
     a. sudden in onset and requires immediate intervention.
     b. easily detected by auscultation.
     c. the result of excessive accumulation of fluid between the pericardium and the myocardium.
     d. characterized by excessive cardiac relaxation, increased blood pressure, and bounding pulse.

14. In the presence of heart failure, which age group is most likely to exhibit liver enlargement before pulmonary edema?
     a. infants
     b. children
     c. adolescents
     d. older adults

15. During cardiac auscultation, the examiner notes a midsystolic murmur with a medium pitch; a coarse thrill is palpated as well. These findings are consistent with which condition?
     a. aortic stenosis
     b. aortic regurgitation
     c. pulmonic stenosis
     d. mitral stenosis

16. Which of the following reports made by a patient suggests compromised cardiac output?
     a. "My heart pounds hard after going upstairs, but it settles down after I rest a minute."
     b. "My right foot hurts a lot. I have also noticed it is colder and darker than the left foot."
     c. "I have been really tired lately. By evening I am too tired to do anything but lie down."
     d. "I keep getting sores on my legs and feet that take forever to heal."

17. Which of the following cardiovascular findings would be considered normal for a woman 8 months pregnant?
     a. The heart position shifts up and to the left; the apex moves laterally.
     b. Percussion reveals a decrease in left ventricular size.
     c. Assessment of the lower legs reveal 3+ pitting edema.
     d. Blood pressure is 150/118.

18. Which principle helps the examiner to determine where heart sounds are best heard?
     a. The Doppler effect diminishes the sound over time.
     b. Sound is transmitted in the direction of blood flow.
     c. Accumulation of fluid magnifies the intensity of sound.
     d. Duration of sound varies directly with frequency.

19. S_2 is:
     a. the result of opening of the atrioventricular valves.
     b. the beginning of systole.
     c. best heard in the mitral area.
     d. of higher pitch and shorter duration than S_1.

Copyright © 2003, Mosby, Inc. All rights reserved.

20. Splitting of heart sounds is:
    a. an unexpected event that should be further evaluated.
    b. the result of opening of the valves during exhalation.
    c. greatest at the peak of inspiration.
    d. due to synchronization of valve closure.

21. To distinguish a murmur from respiratory sounds in an infant, the examiner could correctly do which of the following?
    a. time the sound with the carotid pulsation
    b. distract the child with a moving toy
    c. ask the child to hold his or her breath
    d. use the flat side of the stethoscope to auscultate the child's chest

22. On a young child the examiner notes a systolic ejection murmur that is loud, harsh, and high in pitch heard over the second intercostal space along the left sternal border. What problem should the examiner suspect?
    a. mitral valve prolapse
    b. mitral valve stenosis
    c. coarctation of the aorta
    d. atrial septal defect

23. In order to hear low-pitched filling sounds of the heart, the examiner should place the patient in:
    a. supine position and listen with bell of stethoscope.
    b. a sitting position and listen with the diaphragm of the stethoscope.
    c. a sitting position and listen with the bell of the stethoscope.
    d. a left lateral recumbent position and listen with bell of stethoscope.

24. The heart rates of children:
    a. are less variable than those of adults.
    b. may increase significantly with each degree of temperature elevation.
    c. react slowly to stress of any sort.
    d. tend to increase with age.

25. Common cardiac findings among the elderly include:
    a. vagal tone maintains the heart rate in a narrow range.
    b. cardiac response to demands is rapid and effective.
    c. apical pulse is more difficult to locate.
    d. ectopic beats are usual and signal serious pathology.

Copyright © 2003, Mosby, Inc. All rights reserved.

Terminology Review

Crossword Puzzle

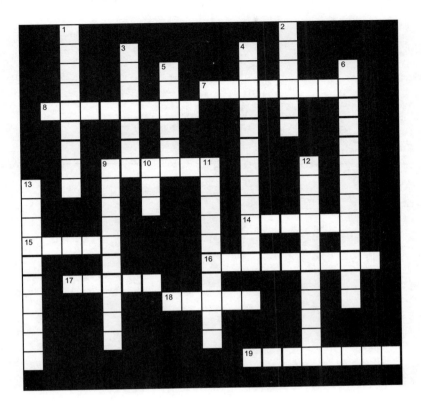

Across

7. Fibers of the ventricular myocardium that conduct the electrical impulses in the heart
8. Phase of cardiac cycle where ventricles dilate
9. Partition dividing left and right heart chambers
14. Substernal pain or intense pressure radiating to neck, jaw, arms
15. Reservoirs for blood returning to heart
16. Fever occurring after streptococcal pharyngitis or skin infection; a systemic connective tissue disease
17. Percentage of increase in blood volume during pregnancy
18. Murmur occurring in healthy children 3 to 7 years of age
19. Valve that separates right ventricle from pulmonary artery

Down

1. Type of electrical conduction system that makes the heart autonomous
2. Fine, palpable, rushing vibration
3. Contraction phase of cardiac cycle
4. Enlargement of right ventricle secondary to pulmonary malfunction
5. Congenital syndrome that is characterized by cyanosis after the neonatal period
6. Backward flow of blood
9. Node where impulse of stimulation originates
10. Where apical pulse is most readily seen or felt
11. Middle layer of the heart; responsible for pumping action
12. Double-walled, fibrous sac encasing the heart
13. Myocardial necrosis secondary to abrupt decrease in coronary blood flow

Copyright © 2003, Mosby, Inc. All rights reserved.

Anatomy Review

On the illustration below, identify the structures of the heart by writing the correct term in the corresponding lettered answer space.

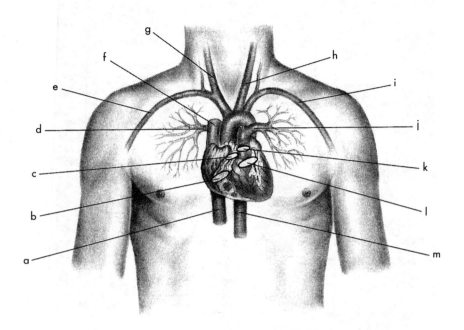

aorta	pulmonic valve
aortic valve	right common carotid artery
inferior vena cava	right pulmonary artery
left common carotid artery	right subclavian artery
left pulmonary artery	superior vena cava
left subclavian artery	tricuspid valve
mitral valve	

a. _____   h. _____

b. _____   i. _____

c. _____   j. _____

d. _____   k. _____

e. _____   l. _____

f. _____   m. _____

g. _____

Copyright © 2003, Mosby, Inc. All rights reserved.

CONCEPTS APPLICATION

Complete the following table by indicating where you would auscultate to locate each.

Valve	Where Would You Auscultate?
Tricuspid valve	
Mitral valve	
Aortic valve	
Pulmonic valve	

CASE STUDY

Howard is a 76-year-old man complaining of difficulty breathing. Listed below are initial data collected during an interview and examination.

Interview Data

Howard doesn't know exactly when his breathing difficulty started, but it has gotten noticeably worse the last couple of days. He volunteers at the church library three mornings a week and plays golf twice a week. However, he tells the examiner that this last week he has "just felt too tired to do anything." Howard says that he has not been able to sleep very well at night because of his breathing difficulty. He adds, "I keep coughing out this frothy-looking phlegm." Howard denies taking any medications at this time. He says that he doesn't smoke or drink alcoholic beverages.

Examination Data

General survey: Alert, cooperative, well-groomed male. Appears stated age. Breathing is mildly labored.

Vital signs: Temperature 98.8° F (37.1° C). Pulse 120. Respirations 26. BP 142/112 right arm; 144/110 left arm.

Pulses: All pulses palpable 2+. No carotid bruits bilaterally.

Lower extremities: Skin warm and dry, without cyanosis. Even hair distribution. 2+ pitting edema noted bilaterally. No lesions present.

Neck: Jugular distension and pulsation noted with patient in supine position.

Copyright © 2003, Mosby, Inc. All rights reserved.

1. What data deviate from normal findings, suggesting a need for further investigation?

2. What additional questions could the nurse ask to clarify symptoms?

3. What additional physical examination, if any, should the nurse complete?

4. What kind of problems do you anticipate this patient will have?

CRITICAL THINKING

1. Mrs. Martin tells you that her 2 1/2-year-old son prefers to squat while watching TV rather than to sit on the couch or floor. What significance does this statement potentially have?

2. A 10-year-old girl is brought to the clinic by her mother. The mother tells the examiner that the girl has been very tired and short of breath, and she has been running a low-grade fever. These symptoms have been getting progressively worse over the last few weeks. The only significant health history is treatment for strep throat last month. What specifically should the examiner focus on to aid in the diagnosis?

3. Mr. Yazzie is a 42-year-old Native American with insulin-dependent diabetes mellitus (IDDM). He is seen in the clinic for a diabetic foot ulcer that does not heal. In what ways does IDDM increase Mr. Yazzie's risk for cardiovascular-related problems?

Copyright © 2003, Mosby, Inc. All rights reserved.

Blood Vessels

LEARNING OBJECTIVES

After studying Chapter 14 in the textbook and completing this section of the workbook, students should be able to:

1. Describe anatomy and physiology of the blood vessels.
2. Identify age and condition variations in the blood vessels.
3. Describe interview questions pertinent to blood vessels examination.
4. Discuss inspection, palpation, percussion, and auscultation techniques for examination of the blood vessels.
5. Describe age-specific and/or condition-specific variations in examination findings of the blood vessels.
6. Identify examination findings associated with various conditions of the blood vessels.

TEXTBOOK REVIEW

Chapter 14   Blood Vessels (pages 462–495)

CONTENT REVIEW QUESTIONS

Multiple Choice

Circle the correct answer for each of the following questions.

1. The carotid artery is considered the most suitable artery for evaluation of cardiac function because it:
   a. is the largest artery in the peripheral vascular system.
   b. is the most pliable artery in the peripheral vascular system.
   c. is the most accessible artery close to the heart.
   d. has the thickest layer of smooth muscle within the vessel walls.

2. The purpose of the great vessels is to:
   a. provide a reservoir for blood volume to be used in times of stress.
   b. circulate the blood to and from the body and the lungs.
   c. quickly and efficiently move blood in and out of the heart.
   d. send blood to the lungs for large-scale reoxygenation.

Copyright © 2003, Mosby, Inc. All rights reserved.

3. The cardiac output is determined by:
    a. multiplying the stroke volume by the heart rate.
    b. subtracting the heart rate from the blood pressure.
    c. dividing the heart rate by the peripheral vascular resistance.
    d. adding the mean arterial pressure from the stroke volume.

4. Pregnant women may experience palmar erythema and spider telangiectasis as a result of:
    a. peripheral vasodilation with decreased vascular resistance.
    b. peripheral vasoconstriction.
    c. increased peripheral resistance.
    d. peripheral vascular resistance with diminished cardiac output.

5. The examiner suspects a patient has deep vein thrombosis. The examiner dorsiflexes the patient's foot, to which the patient reports calf pain. This finding is referred to as a positive:
    a. Allis' sign.
    b. Chadwick's sign.
    c. Homan's sign.
    d. Kehr's sign.

6. Dilation and tortuosity of the aorta and carotid arteries in elderly patients may be caused by:
    a. calcification of the walls of the arteries.
    b. cholesterol deposits on the walls of the arteries.
    c. postural hypotension.
    d. increased peripheral vascular resistance.

7. Atherosclerosis, anemia, anxiety, and exercise are associated most with which type of arterial pulse?
    a. alternating pulse
    b. bounding pulse
    c. labile pulse
    d. paradoxic pulse

8. Which word best describes a 3+ amplitude pulse?
    a. diminished
    b. normal
    c. full
    d. bounding

9. When evaluating a bruit, which of the following principles is true?
    a. Complete obstruction results in a muffled sound.
    b. Increasing obstruction produces lower pitches.
    c. Mild obstruction produces a short, localized sound.
    d. Sounds due to vigorous left ventricular ejection are more common in adults than children.

10. An arterial aneurysm is most commonly detected by:
    a. palpating the dilation of the artery.
    b. auscultating a bruit over the aneurysm.
    c. percussing a thrill over the aneurysm.
    d. observing redness and swelling over the aneurysm.

11. Claudication is:
    a. tissue necrosis due to venous insufficiency.
    b. pain that results from muscle ischemia.
    c. characterized by sharp, tingling pain.
    d. occurs after exercise and during sleep.

Copyright © 2003, Mosby, Inc. All rights reserved.

12. Korotkoff's sounds:
    a. are best heard with the diaphragm of the stethoscope.
    b. begin with the end of diastole and end at the beginning of systole.
    c. are produced by turbulence of blood flow in an artery.
    d. occur within the auscultatory gap.

13. To determine pulse pressure the examiner would correctly do which of the following?
    a. add the systolic and diastolic readings
    b. palpate the radial pulse while occluding circulation with the blood pressure cuff
    c. subtract the diastolic from the systolic readings
    d. apply manual pressure on the brachial artery while auscultating the Korotkoff's sounds

14. Reliable indicators of hypertension are:
    a. numerous measurements taken over a period of time.
    b. any readings of blood pressure where the systolic pressure exceeds 120 mm Hg.
    c. sitting, standing, and supine readings of blood pressure.
    d. findings of diastolic blood pressure in excess of 80 mm Hg.

15. Postural hypotension should be evaluated in which of the following patients?
    a. an elderly woman taking antihypertensive medication
    b. a pregnant woman with increased plasma volume
    c. all children under the age of 6 years
    d. a middle-aged male complaining of sudden onset of chest pain

16. In determining the jugular venous pressure the examiner would correctly do which of the following?
    a. apply manual pressure on the carotid artery while the patient forcefully exhales
    b. examine neck veins while occluding the brachial artery with the blood pressure cuff
    c. use light to supply tangential illumination across the neck
    d. have the patient lean forward from the waist and take a deep breath

17. Varicose veins are characterized by:
    a. dilation and tortuosity when the extremities are dependant.
    b. increased rate of blood flow to extremities.
    c. decreased intravenous pressure.
    d. edema resulting from obstruction to a distal vein.

18. A condition that results in progressive ischemia caused by insufficient perfusion is:
    a. Raynaud's phenomenon.
    b. peripheral atherosclerotic disease.
    c. venous thrombosis.
    d. arterial aneurysm.

19. In which group is a jugular venous hum an expected examination finding?
    a. older adults
    b. pregnant women
    c. Native Americans
    d. children

20. The patient tells the examiner, "My left leg has been hurting a lot lately, especially when I move my foot up and down. It also seems more swollen then the other leg." Based on the symptoms, the examiner should suspect:
    a. hypertension.
    b. venous stenosis.
    c. venous thrombosis.
    d. arterial insufficiency.

Copyright © 2003, Mosby, Inc. All rights reserved.

21. The examiner notes a prominent jugular vein with significant pulsations. These findings are consistent with:
    a. right-sided heart failure.
    b. hypertension.
    c. cardiac ischemia.
    d. left ventricular hypertrophy.

22. Which test is correctly used to evaluate venous incompetence when varicosities are present?
    a. Rinne
    b. Perthes
    c. Romberg
    d. Trendelenburg

23. The most common cause of venous thrombosis in children is:
    a. congenital venous incompetence.
    b. atherosclerosis of deep veins.
    c. arteriovenous malformation.
    d. placement of venous access devices.

24. Hypertension in children is most often the result of:
    a. Addison's disease.
    b. renal disease.
    c. stress and anxiety.
    d. side effects of prescription medications.

25. Which of the following distinguishes musculoskeletal pain from vascular insufficiency?
    a. onset during activity
    b. increases with intensity and duration of activity
    c. may occur several hours after activity
    d. quickly relieved by rest

Copyright © 2003, Mosby, Inc. All rights reserved.

Terminology Review

Crossword Puzzle

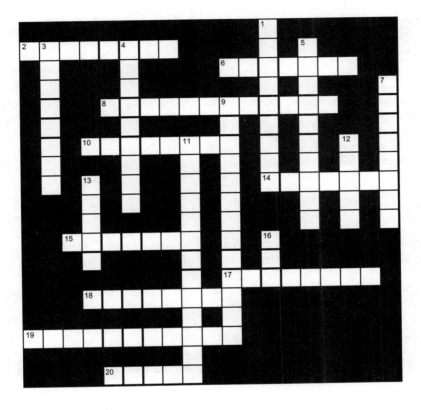

Across

2. Type of veins characterized by dilation and tortuosity
6. Test used to evaluate patency of deep veins
8. Pain resulting from muscle ischemia
10. Type of hypotension which occurs when patient stands up relatively suddenly
14. Type of pathologic communication between an artery and a vein
15. Type of edema characterized by depression that does not rapidly refill and resume original contour
17. Arteritis characterized by flu-like symptoms
18. Disease typified by systemic vasculitis, strawberry tongue, and edema of the hands and feet
19. Congenital aortic stenosis
20. Sign indicating thrombosis in lower extremity

Down

1. Sounds resulting from turbulence of blood flow in an artery
3. Localized dilation of an artery caused by weakness in the vessel wall
4. Condition characterized by pain, pallor, and pulselessness
5. Clotting within a blood vessel which may cause infarction of tissues supplied by the vessel
7. Effect on blood pressure of decreased elasticity of the blood vessels in the elderly
9. Common cause of arterial dilation and tortuosity in the elderly
11. Backflow of blood as a result of incompetent valves
12. Technique used to estimate blood pressure on a child
13. Harsh or musical intermittent auscultatory sound, especially an abnormal one
16. Venous phenomenon common in children and without pathologic significance

Copyright © 2003, Mosby, Inc. All rights reserved.

CASE STUDY

Felice is a 32-year-old woman complaining of pain in her fingers, with more discomfort in the dominant right hand. Listed below are initial data collected during an interview and examination.

Interview Data

Felice began to notice changes in her hands about 3 months ago when she started a new job where she spends several hours a day at a computer keyboard. The pain has steadily increased since then and she is alarmed about the development of a dark spot on the tip of her fifth finger of her right hand. She attends aerobic classes weekly but is not able to keep up with the class due to shortness of breath. She has smoked a pack of cigarettes daily for the last 10 years. She has a moderate alcohol intake of two to three glasses of wine per week. She is taking no medications at this time.

Examination Data

General Survey: Alert, cooperative, well-groomed female who appears stated age. Shortness of breath noted upon reaching the examination room, but abated after one minute of rest.

Vital signs: Temperature 98.8° F (37.1° C). Pulse 100 on arrival to room; 76 after five minutes. BP 126/82 in both arms.

Pulses: All pulses palpable 2+. Fingers on both hands are cool to touch.

Lower extremities: Skin warm and dry, free of cyanosis or erythema. Hair distribution is even. No edema noted. No lesions present.

Upper extremities: Fingers cool, capillary refill sluggish. Noted dark lesion on tip of right fifth finger 4 mm diameter. Some reduced range of motion noted in both hands. The skin over the hands appears tight and probably contributed to the reduced range of motion.

Neck: Supple. No neck vein distention noted.

1. What data deviate from normal findings, suggesting a need for further investigation?

2. What additional questions could the examiner ask to clarify symptoms?

Copyright © 2003, Mosby, Inc. All rights reserved.

3. What additional physical examination, if any, should the examiner complete?

4. What kind of problems do you anticipate this patient will have?

CRITICAL THINKING

1. Mr. Simmons reports that he has increasing pain in the calf of his left leg which he began to notice following a long airplane ride 1 month ago. He is 56 years old and has smoked a half a pack of cigarettes a day for the last 20 years. Examination reveals some redness and tenderness over the affected area. What do his symptoms suggest and what is he at risk for?

2. Mrs. Porter comes to her routine prenatal check at 32 weeks complaining of difficulty with dizziness when she gets up from bed or from a seated position. What is the most likely cause for her symptoms?

Copyright © 2003, Mosby, Inc. All rights reserved.

15

Breasts and Axillae

LEARNING OBJECTIVES

After studying Chapter 14 in the textbook and completing this section of the workbook, students should be able to:

1. Conduct a history related to the breasts and axillae.
2. Discuss examination techniques for the breasts and axillae.
3. Identify normal age and condition variations to the breasts and axillae.
4. Recognize findings that deviate from expected findings.
5. Relate symptoms or clinical findings to common pathologic conditions.

TEXTBOOK REVIEW

Chapter 15   Breasts and Axillae (pages 496–524)

CONTENT REVIEW QUESTIONS

Multiple Choice

Circle the correct answer for each of the following questions.

1. A patient complains of a red rash on her breast. Which finding helps an examiner differentiate Paget's disease from eczema? The lesion is:
   a. unilateral.
   b. red.
   c. located on the nipple.
   d. raised and fluid-filled.

Copyright © 2003, Mosby, Inc. All rights reserved.

2. Yvonne had a mastectomy to the right breast 2 years ago. Which true statement assists the examiner with breast examination of this patient?
    a. Swelling, thickening, and small lumps around the mastectomy site are normal.
    b. The mastectomy site should be inspected but not palpated because of pain at the site.
    c. If malignancy recurs, it may be at the scar site.
    d. There is no need to examine the mastectomy site.

3. A women in her third trimester of pregnancy asks the examiner about the drainage from her nipples. Her nipples are symmetric without redness. Which statement is true?
    a. Colostrum secretion is normal in the last trimester.
    b. Cultures should be taken to rule out an infection.
    c. Drainage from the nipple is an indication of a malignancy.
    d. The drainage is a sign of witch's milk.

4. While palpating the axilla, it is best to place the patient in a:
    a. sitting position with hands over head.
    b. sitting position with arms at sides.
    c. supine position with arms on hips.
    d. lateral position with arms at sides.

5. A 58-year-old woman asks the examiner how often a mammogram is recommended for her. The best response by the examiner is:
    a. "every 1 to 2 years if you have no symptoms."
    b. "every 3 years."
    c. "every 5 years if you have no symptoms."
    d. "every 3 years if you have a family history of cancer."

6. A supernumerary nipple is found on a Caucasian newborn infant girl. Which of the following may accompany this finding?
    a. increased risk for breast cancer as an adult
    b. increased lactation volume as an adult
    c. congenital renal or cardiac anomalies
    d. mental retardation

7. A patient reports that she is concerned about the changes in her breasts that accompany her menstrual cycle. What should the examiner tell her about these changes?
    a. These changes are most likely to occur prior to and after the menstrual flow.
    b. These changes are alarming and might signal the development of a malignancy.
    c. These changes are a common response to hormonal changes during the menstrual cycle.
    d. Changes are most noticeable during the week after menstrual flow.

8. Which of the following is the correct position in which to place the patient for breast palpation?
    a. supine with arms at side; pillow under neck
    b. supine with arm over head and small pillow under shoulder of side being assessed
    c. left lateral position with arm bent backward
    d. sitting slightly forward with breasts hanging away from chest; hands on hips

9. Which statement made by a 37-year-old woman would make the examiner suspect fibrocystic disease?
    a. "I have a lump in my breast that is not tender."
    b. "My right breast is larger than the left breast."
    c. "My nipples are darker than before my baby was born."
    d. "I feel a lump before my period."

Copyright © 2003, Mosby, Inc. All rights reserved.

10. A patient, 3 weeks postpartum, tells the examiner that she is breast-feeding, but might stop because her nipples are sore. The examiner observes dry and cracked nipples. Which of the following questions would be helpful in gaining information relevant to treating the problem?
    a. "Do you pump your breasts?"
    b. "How do you clean your breasts?"
    c. "Have you been able to bond with your infant?"
    d. "What medications have you been taking?"

11. In an older male, gynecomastia may be secondary to:
    a. a decrease in physical activity.
    b. increased lactiferous duct glands.
    c. lymphatic engorgement.
    d. a decrease in testosterone.

12. Which of the following questions asked by the examiner will best validate the patient's understanding of breast self-examination?
    a. "Do you do breast examinations on yourself?"
    b. "How often do you examine your breasts?"
    c. "Would you show me how you examine your breasts?"
    d. "Why is breast self-examination important to do on a regular basis?"

13. Symptoms consistent with underlying ductal malignancy include:
    a. erythema, heat, and pain over and around one nipple.
    b. red, scaling, crusty patch on one nipple.
    c. bilateral inflammation, tenderness, and sticky multicolored nipple discharge.
    d. gynecomastia and a deepening color of the nipple.

14. While examining the breast of a 52-year-old woman, the examiner notes nipple discharge. Which of the following diagnostic tests would be appropriate?
    a. cytologic examination of the discharge
    b. culture and sensitivity examination of the discharge
    c. white blood cell count
    d. estrogen level

15. While performing a breast examination on a 68-year-old female, which finding is expected? The:
    a. breast tissue has multiple large, firm lumps in it.
    b. breast tissue has a granular feel to it.
    c. tail of Spence is no longer observed.
    d. axillary lymph nodes are enlarged.

Terminology Review

Matching

Match each clinical finding to its corresponding associated factor or cause.

Clinical Finding	Associated Factor or Cause
16. _____ Galactorrhea	a. Malignant breast tumor
17. _____ Mastitis	b. Ductal enlargement
18. _____ Fibrocystic disease	c. Possible sign of breast malignancy
19. _____ Dimpling in breast	d. Administration of phenothiazines
20. _____ Nipple retraction	e. Clogged milk duct

Copyright © 2003, Mosby, Inc. All rights reserved.

Crossword Puzzle

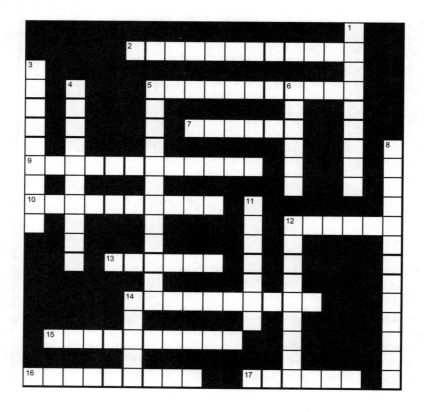

Across

2. Unexpected enlargement of breast tissue
5. Disease resulting in benign breast cyst formation
7. Projection at the apex of the breast on the surface of which the lactiferous ducts open
9. Lactation not associated with child-bearing
10. Important constituent of colostrum in addition to protein and minerals
12. Staging for sexual maturity
13. Ligaments that support the breast
14. Small tumors of the subareolar ducts
15. Follicles that are tiny sebaceous glands and may appear in the areola
16. Clear or milky white fluid expressed from breast prior to milk production
17. Pigmented area surrounding the nipple

Down

1. Peau d'orange appearance indicates blocked lymph drainage in this condition
3. Common radiologic procedure for breast examination
4. Interval following termination of lactation when breasts decrease in size
5. Benign neoplasm of breast tissue
6. Area where most malignancies occur in breast tissue
8. Exceeding the normal number
11. Lymph nodes signaling lymphatic invasion of carcinoma from abdomen or thorax
12. Beginning of breast development in the female
14. Disease which is a surface manifestation of underlying ductal carcinoma

Copyright © 2003, Mosby, Inc. All rights reserved.

CONCEPTS APPLICATION

On the illustrations below, draw the direction of palpation the examiner would use for (a) back-and-forth technique; (b) concentric circles technique; and (c) wedge technique.

a

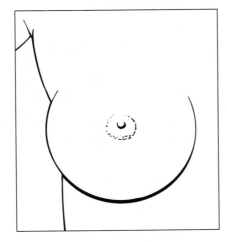

b

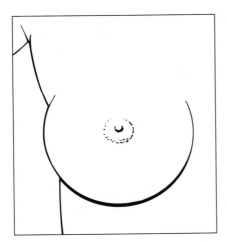

c

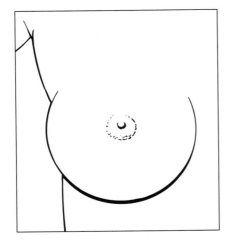

Copyright © 2003, Mosby, Inc. All rights reserved.

CASE STUDY

Julie is a 46-year-old female who comes to the clinic because she has discovered a lump in her left breast. Listed below are data collected during an interview and examination.

Interview Data

Julie tells the examiner that she first noticed the lump about 9 months ago. Because it seemed small and did not hurt, she did not feel that it was much to worry about. Recently, Julie began noticing that the lump felt bigger and decided she better have someone look at it. Julie tells the examiner, "I just know it is not cancer because I am much too young and healthy. And if it is, I am not about to let some doctor mutilate me with a knife. I'd rather die than have my breast cut off." The examiner asks her if she has noticed any redness or dimpling of the breast. Julie tells the examiner, "No, not really, but I don't pay attention to those sorts of things." Julie tells the examiner that she started having regular menstrual cycles at the age of 11 and still has not reached menopause. She has never been married and has no children.

Examination Data

General survey: Very nervous, well-nourished female. Is hesitant to expose her breast for examination.

Breast exam: Inspection reveals breasts of typical size with right and left breast symmetry. The skin of both breasts is smooth, with even pigmentation. The nipples protrude slightly with no drainage noted. The left nipple is slightly retracted. Significant dimpling noted on left breast in upper outer quadrant when arms are raised over her head. Right breast appears normal. Palpation of the left breast reveals a large hard lump in the upper outer quadrant. No lumps or masses noted in right breast. The left nipple produces a clear bloody-type discharge when squeezed; the right nipple is unremarkable.

1. What data deviate from normal findings, suggesting a need for further investigation?

2. What additional questions could the examiner ask to clarify symptoms?

3. What additional physical examination, if any, should the examiner complete?

4. What primary problems does the patient have?

Copyright © 2003, Mosby, Inc. All rights reserved.

CRITICAL THINKING

1. A 43-year-old female patient tells you her mother died of breast cancer and her 50-year-old sister currently has breast cancer. She is worried about developing breast cancer as well. Her gynecologic history includes menarche at age 11. She has one child, a 7-year-old son. She has no history of other pregnancies and no history of illness. List her current risk factors. Would you consider her to be at high risk for breast cancer?

2. A 23-year-old female requests information on how to perform breast self-examination. Describe essential elements you would want to include in a teaching plan.

Copyright © 2003, Mosby, Inc. All rights reserved.

16

Abdomen

LEARNING OBJECTIVES

After studying Chapter 16 in the textbook and completing this section of the workbook, students should be able to:

1. Conduct a history related to the abdomen.
2. Discuss examination techniques for the abdomen.
3. Identify normal age and condition variations of the abdomen.
4. Recognize findings that deviate from expected findings.
5. Relate symptoms or clinical findings to common pathologic conditions.

TEXTBOOK REVIEW

Chapter 16   Abdomen (pages 525–583)

CONTENT REVIEW QUESTIONS

Multiple Choice

Circle the correct answer for each of the following questions.

1. Which statement made by a patient suggests that the patient has a risk for viral hepatitis A? "I:
   a. am a health care worker."
   b. had a blood transfusion recently."
   c. have renal failure and have hemodialysis three times a week."
   d. have recently been overseas."

2. The examiner observes venous return on the abdomen of the patient that moves upward from the pubis to the chest. This finding should make the examiner consider:
   a. portal hypertension.
   b. renal artery stenosis.
   c. inferior vena cava obstruction.
   d. mesentery artery hypertension.

Copyright © 2003, Mosby, Inc. All rights reserved.   **123**

3. Which of the following questions would help an examiner determine whether a patient has an intra-abdominal infection?
    a. "Where is the pain?"
    b. "Would you like something to eat?"
    c. "What does your urine look like?"
    d. "Is there a history of this problem in your family?"

4. Mrs. Cody is 36 weeks pregnant. She tells the examiner she feels like her stomach muscle is splitting. A light protrusion of the abdomen midline is observed. This is recognized as:
    a. abdominal dehiscence.
    b. swelling of the abdominal aorta.
    c. diastasis recti.
    d. umbilical herniation.

5. In which of the following patients would a slight pulsation in the epigastric area be considered a normal inspection finding?
    a. a very thin patient
    b. an obese patient
    c. a patient with ascites
    d. an elderly patient

6. The examiner palpates an organ in the left costal margin. Which technique should the examiner use to differentiate between an enlarged left kidney and an enlarged spleen?
    a. auscultation, listening for renal bruit
    b. auscultation, listening for abdominal friction rub
    c. palpation, using indirect fist palpation to assess for tenderness
    d. percussion, listening for dullness

7. A hiatal hernia is best described as:
    a. a protrusion of abdominal contents through a weakening in the abdominal wall.
    b. a protrusion of the stomach through the esophageal hiatus of the diaphragm.
    c. an ulcer in the mucosa of the stomach that herniates into the peritoneal cavity.
    d. a herniation of the gallbladder into the cystic duct.

8. An examiner may wish to use a bimanual technique for abdominal palpation when:
    a. palpating superficial organs.
    b. validating abdominal tenderness in the infant.
    c. meeting muscle resistance while performing deep palpation.
    d. determining the presence of excessive peritoneal fluid.

9. Fetal well-being can be assessed by fetal heart rate and:
    a. adequate maternal weight gain.
    b. fetal position.
    c. measurement of abdominal girth.
    d. kick count.

10. A history of chest pain is collected as part of an abdominal history because it may be:
    a. associated with ulcers.
    b. caused by esophageal herniation and edema.
    c. perceived as esophagus and stomach pain.
    d. related to congenital abdominal defects.

Copyright © 2003, Mosby, Inc. All rights reserved.

11. The examiner lightly stokes each quadrant of the abdomen with the end of a reflex hammer by stroking outwards from the navel. Which of the following describes the expected finding?
    a. contraction of the abdominal muscle, pulling of the umbilicus toward the stroked side
    b. contraction of the abdominal muscle, pulling of the umbilicus away from the stroked side
    c. rippling motion of the abdomen associated with peristaltic activity
    d. absence of abdominal movement

12. How is fundal height measured? Measure from the:
    a. umbilicus to the top of the fundus.
    b. perineum to the top of the fundus.
    c. symphysis pubis to the top of the fundus.
    d. xyphoid process to the top of the fundus.

13. You note that the midclavicular liver span of an adult male patient is 18 cm. With palpation you note that the liver is enlarged, hard, and nontender. What do these findings suggest?
    a. diverticulitis
    b. ulcerative colitis
    c. hepatitis
    d. cirrhosis

14. The examiner is unable to palpate the liver or kidney on the patient. Which of the following techniques will help assess tenderness to these organs?
    a. direct, continuous, firm pressure over the organ for several minutes
    b. percussion for tympany
    c. percussion for size
    d. indirect fist percussion

15. In which age group does abdominal palpation become easier and more accurate?
    a. young children
    b. adolescents
    c. young adults
    d. older adults

16. Which of the following techniques is used to confirm the presence of abdominal ascites?
    a. auscultation of fluid movement within the abdominal cavity
    b. palpation of rebound tenderness
    c. palpation of pitting edema on the abdomen
    d. percussion of dullness over dependent areas of the abdomen

17. A 5-week-old male infant is brought to the clinic with a 2-day history of projectile vomiting. What specific finding should the examiner assess for?
    a. abdominal pain with palpation
    b. palpation of small, round mass
    c. auscultation of tinkering bowel sounds
    d. auscultation of bruit over renal artery

18. Which of the following examination findings is indicative of peritoneal irritation or appendicitis?
    a. palpation of rebound tenderness
    b. percussion of shifting dullness over the abdomen
    c. auscultation of a bruit over the abdominal aorta
    d. percussion of dullness over the suprapubic area

Copyright © 2003, Mosby, Inc. All rights reserved.

19. Fetal movement (quickening) is determined through which examination technique?
    a. auscultation—hearing the fetal movement within uterus
    b. palpation—by placing a hand over the abdomen
    c. deep palpation—feeling fetal movement as you push your hand against abdomen
    d. percussion—noting changes in tone as the fetus moves in the uterus

20. Which finding on a newborn infant suggests a congenital anomaly?
    a. The umbilical cord has one artery and one vein.
    b. The umbilical cord is thick.
    c. The umbilical cord is thin.
    d. There is a small mass around the umbilicus.

21. A 32-year-old female patient tells the examiner that when she goes running, she dribbles urine. Which type of problem should the examiner consider?
    a. hydronephrosis
    b. renal abscess
    c. stress incontinence
    d. overflow incontinence

22. A 61-year-old man has a presenting complaint of frequent constipation. He tells the examiner that there has been a change in his bowel movement habits—he gets constipated easily, the stool is very "skinny-looking," and it is a different color than usual. He denies pain. What do these symptoms suggest?
    a. diverticulitis
    b. hepatitis B
    c. colon or rectal cancer
    d. pancreatitis

23. The functional ability of the GI tract most severely affected by aging is:
    a. motility.
    b. metabolism.
    c. digestion.
    d. catabolism.

24. What is the correct name of the rule that states that the farther away from the navel abdominal pain occurs, the more likely it is to be of physical importance?
    a. Reglan rule
    b. Appley rule
    c. Applegate rule
    d. Romberg rule

25. Which of the following signs is an absence of bowel sounds in the right lower quadrant which indicates the possibility of intussusception?
    a. Grey Turner
    b. Aaron
    c. Dance
    d. Markle

Copyright © 2003, Mosby, Inc. All rights reserved.

Terminology Review

Matching

Match each clinical finding to its corresponding abdominal condition.

Clinical Finding

26. _____ Knifelike pain
27. _____ Dark yellow urine
28. _____ Pain with gradual onset
29. _____ Colic pain
30. _____ Bruit
31. _____ Burning pain

Abdominal Condition

a. Intra-abdominal infectious process
b. Ulcer
c. Liver/biliary disease
d. Pancreatitis
e. Renal stone
f. Aortic aneurysm

Crossword Puzzle

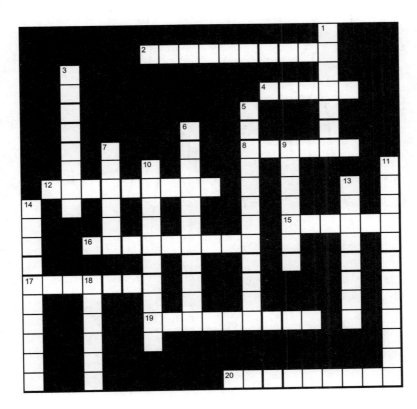

Across

2. Excessive quantity of amniotic fluid
4. Spasmodic pains in the abdomen
8. Enzyme that acts on emulsified fats
12. Destruction of liver parenchyma
15. Backflow caused by relaxation or incompetence of lower esophagus
16. Sound obtained on percussing a part that can vibrate freely
17. Low-pitched, resonant, drumlike note obtained by percussing the surface of a large, air-containing space
19. Fan-shaped fold of peritoneum that anchors small intestine to abdominal wall
20. Inflammatory process of liver, usually caused by viral infection

Down

1. Accumulation of serous fluid in the peritoneal cavity
3. Abdomen that suggests diaphragmatic hernia in the newborn
5. Palpation technique used to assess a floating mass
6. Muscular contractions that move products of digestion through the alimentary canal
7. Commonly known as "stretch marks"
9. Distal section of the stomach
10. Rumbling or gurgling noises produced by movement of gas in the alimentary canal
11. Uterine contractions that may begin in the first trimester
13. Twisting of the intestine resulting in an obstruction
14. Serous membrane lining the abdominal cavity
18. Enzyme that acts to digest proteins

Copyright © 2003, Mosby, Inc. All rights reserved.

Anatomy Review

Activity 1

On the illustration below, identify the structures of the abdomen by writing the correct term in the corresponding lettered answer space. Use each term once.

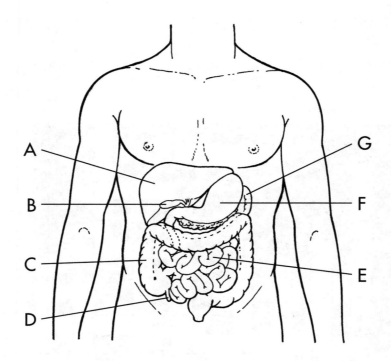

appendix	pancreas
colon	small intestine
gallbladder	spleen
liver	stomach

a. _____   e. _____

b. _____   f. _____

c. _____   g. _____

d. _____   h. _____

Copyright © 2003, Mosby, Inc. All rights reserved.

Activity 2

Consider the two recognized divisions of the abdomen: four quadrants of the abdomen and nine regions of the abdomen, found on page XXX of the textbook. Referring to the illustration in Activity 1, identify on the chart below the quadrant and the region where each of the listed abdominal structures are located. (Some structures are found in more than one quadrant or region.) The first one has been done for you.

Structure	Quadrant	Region
Appendix	right lower quadrant	right inguinal
Colon		
Gallbladder		
Liver		
Pancreas		
Small intestine		
Spleen		
Stomach		

Copyright © 2003, Mosby, Inc. All rights reserved.

CONCEPTS APPLICATION

Complete the table below to compare and contrast types of pain, abdominal signs, and associated symptoms or findings of the various conditions.

Condition	Type of Pain	Abdominal Signs or Findings	Associated Symptoms
Peritonitis	Sudden or gradual onset of generalized or localized pain described as dull or severe; increased pain with deep inspiration		
		+ Murphy sign	
Ectopic pregnancy			Tender cervix, discharge, dyspareunia
	Sudden and dramatic LUQ, umbilical, or epigastric pain that may be referred to L shoulder		Fever, epigastric tenderness, vomiting
		+ Kehr sign	Fever, hematuria

Copyright © 2003, Mosby, Inc. All rights reserved.

CASE STUDY

Katie is an 18-year-old female complaining of abdominal pain. Listed below are data collected by the examiner during an interview and examination.

Interview Data

Katie tells the examiner the pain started yesterday evening and has gotten progressively worse. She describes the pain as "really bad." The pain is constant and located in her right lower abdomen, toward her umbilicus. She says that her pain feels a little better if she stays curled up and does not move. She tells the examiner that she is in good health and that she has never had a problem with her stomach. Katie indicates that normally she has a good appetite and can eat anything . . . except for now. She says she ate breakfast and lunch yesterday, but by dinnertime she was nauseated and had no appetite. She has not eaten anything since. She has had no recent weight changes, but she would like to weigh about 5 pounds less than she currently does. Katie does not smoke or drink alcoholic beverages, and she takes no medication. She denies discomfort or problems with urination, describing her urine as "usual-looking."

Examination Data

General survey: Alert and anxious female in moderate distress lying in a fetal position on the examination table, with her eyes closed. Appears well-nourished but not obese. Her skin is hot.

Abdominal inspection: Abdomen is flat and symmetric. No lesions or scars noted. No surface movements are seen except for breathing.

Abdominal auscultation: Bowel sounds absent.

Abdominal percussion: Tympany noted over most of abdominal surface; dullness over liver. Midclavicular liver span is 4 inches.

Light abdominal palpation: Demonstrates pain and guarding in right lower quadrant. Unable to palpate deep structures because of excessive abdominal discomfort. Demonstrates positive rebound tenderness in right lower quadrant.

1. What data deviate from normal findings, suggesting a need for further investigation?

2. What additional questions could the examiner ask to clarify symptoms?

Copyright © 2003, Mosby, Inc. All rights reserved.

3. What additional physical examination, if any, should the examiner complete?

4. What primary problems does the patient have?

CRITICAL THINKING

1. As you auscultate the abdomen, you should listen not only for bowel sounds, but vascular sounds and a friction rub as well. List specifically what you are listening to and what abnormal findings may indicate.

2. Mr. Cane is a 46-year-old male with liver cirrhosis. You are preparing to check for ascites using a fluid wave technique. How is this particular procedure done, and what is a positive finding?

3. Cindy is a 24-year-old female who is 7 months pregnant. Describe expected findings during an abdominal examination that are unique to pregnancy.

Copyright © 2003, Mosby, Inc. All rights reserved.

Female Genitalia

LEARNING OBJECTIVES

After studying Chapter 17 in the textbook and completing this section of the workbook, students should be able to:

1. Conduct a history related to the female genitalia.
2. Discuss examination techniques for the female genitalia.
3. Identify normal age and condition variations of the female genitalia.
4. Recognize findings that deviate from expected findings.
5. Relate symptoms or clinical findings to common pathologic conditions.

TEXTBOOK REVIEW

Chapter 17   Female Genitalia (pages 584–647)

CONTENT REVIEW QUESTIONS

Multiple Choice

Circle the correct answer for each of the following questions.

1. Which finding is suggestive of pelvic inflammatory disease?
   a. enlargement of ovaries
   b. everted cervix
   c. pain resulting from movement of cervix
   d. unilateral labial swelling, redness, and tenderness

2. Which finding would be of concern during an examination of an elderly female patient?
   a. palpable ovaries
   b. small and pale cervix
   c. constriction of the vaginal introitus
   d. absence of vaginal rugation

Copyright © 2003, Mosby, Inc. All rights reserved.

3. While palpating the introitus of the vagina, the patient jumps and complains of severe tenderness. A mass is palpated that is warm to touch. Which of the following problems are these clinical findings consistent with?
   a. cancer of the cervix
   b. inflammation of the Bartholin's glands
   c. a cystocele
   d. acute genital wart infection

4. Which finding may be indicative of a pelvic mass? The cervix is:
   a. pale in color.
   b. deviating to the right.
   c. protruding 2.5 cm into the vagina.
   d. pointing anteriorly.

5. The vagina, uterus, fallopian tubes, and ovaries are supported by four ligaments. Which of the following is a normal examination finding that evaluates this support? The:
   a. uterus can be moved back and forth with manipulation.
   b. patient is able to tolerate a wide-blade speculum during examination.
   c. uterus and ovaries are easily assessed with bimanual palpation.
   d. vagina and uterus are fixed and do not move with manipulation.

6. Which information is accurate and appropriate for an examiner to share with the patient following a Pap smear?
   a. "You may have heavier bleeding with your next menstrual period."
   b. "You may experience abdominal cramping for the next couple of days."
   c. "You will feel nauseated for the rest of the day."
   d. "You may experience mild bleeding or spotting over the next couple of hours."

7. A patient complains of pain, dysmenorrhea, and heavy prolonged menstrual flow. Tender nodules are palpable along the uterosacral ligament. The symptoms and findings suggest:
   a. pelvic inflammatory disease.
   b. endometriosis.
   c. ectopic pregnancy.
   d. ovarian cancer.

8. An examiner plans to collect samples for cytologic studies during a vaginal examination. Prior to the examination, the examiner should lubricate the speculum with:
   a. a water-soluble lubricant.
   b. topical anesthetizing ointment.
   c. warm water.
   d. vaginal secretions.

9. Symptoms associated with PMS are caused by:
   a. ovulation.
   b. thickening of the uterine lining.
   c. elevations in body temperature.
   d. fluctuations in hormone levels.

10. When examining a woman who has had a hysterectomy, the examiner should:
    a. delete the bimanual and palpation maneuvers.
    b. obtain a Pap smear from the suture line.
    c. omit cultures and specimens from the vagina.
    d. palpate internal areas before inserting the speculum.

Copyright © 2003, Mosby, Inc. All rights reserved.

11. A patient complains of urinary incontinence when she is active. Which associated finding might explain this problem?
    a. hernial protrusion in the posterior wall of the vagina
    b. hernial protrusion through the anterior wall of the vagina
    c. symptoms associated with PMS
    d. enlargement and protrusion of the cervix into the vaginal vault

12. Which finding suggests an infection with a sexually transmitted disease?
    a. ulcers and vesicles on the vulva
    b. atrophy of labia minora
    c. dilation of the urethral orifice
    d. bluish color to the cervix

13. The examiner observes a slit-shaped cervical os in a nulliparous woman. Which of the following data in her history explains this finding? The patient:
    a. had early onset of menarche.
    b. has had multiple sex partners.
    c. has had infection with the human papilloma virus (HPV).
    d. had an abortion as a teenager.

14. A prominent labia minora in a newborn:
    a. indicates a maternal infection.
    b. suggests ambiguous genitalia.
    c. is consistent with prematurity.
    d. is a normal finding.

15. The mother of a 6-year-old girl expresses concern that her daughter seems to be experiencing vaginal bleeding. Which statement regarding vaginal bleeding in children is true?
    a. Vaginal bleeding in children is always a sign of sexual abuse.
    b. Vaginal bleeding in children is always clinically important.
    c. Vaginal bleeding in children is most commonly caused by carcinoma of the cervix.
    d. Occasional vaginal bleeding in the child is considered a benign finding.

16. Softness of the cervix is an expected finding for:
    a. an adolescent.
    b. a pregnant woman.
    c. a nonpregnant woman.
    d. an older adult.

17. In what way is the pelvic outlet estimated on a pregnant patient?
    a. Insert a speculum into the patient's vagina and open as widely as possible. Measure the distance between the two blades.
    b. Insert two fingers into the vagina until fingers touch the cervix. Measure the distance to the cervix.
    c. Place the palm of the hand over the perineum, spread fingers to the width of the ischial tuberosities, and measure.
    d. Use a Thom pelvimeter to measure the bi-ischial diameter.

18. A cauliflower-like mass found on the labia of a female patient is most likely caused by:
    a. primary syphilis.
    b. condyloma latum.
    c. condyloma acuminatum.
    d. venereal herpes.

Copyright © 2003, Mosby, Inc. All rights reserved.

19. A sexually active, single, 22-year-old patient complains of a "gross" vaginal discharge. Which of the following questions helps the examiner understand this symptom?
    a. "Do you use condoms?"
    b. "What type of oral contraceptives do you take?"
    c. "At what age did you start menstruating?"
    d. "Do you have a family history of ovarian or breast cancer?"

20. A 62-year-old female patient went through menopause about 14 years ago. Which statement made by this patient indicates a need for further follow-up?
    a. "I have not been sexually active for about 4 years."
    b. "My pubic hair has become very thin."
    c. "I have small amounts of vaginal bleeding a couple of times a week."
    d. "I have been taking extra calcium since I reached menopause."

Terminology Review

Matching

Match each type of malignancy to its corresponding risk factors. Some risk factors have more than one answer.

Risk Factor

21. _____ History of breast cancer
22. _____ Smoking
23. _____ Infertility or nulliparity
24. _____ High socioeconomic status
25. _____ Multiple pregnancies
26. _____ Age 46
27. _____ Multiple sex partners
28. _____ Early menarche
29. _____ Obesity
30. _____ Infection with human papilloma virus

Malignancy

O: ovarian cancer
C: cervical cancer
E: endometrial cancer

Match each diagnostic lab test to the type of instrument used to collect the specimen.

Diagnostic Test

31. _____ Gonococcal culture
32. _____ Endocervical cells
33. _____ DNA probe for chlamydia and gonorrhea
34. _____ *Trichomonas vaginalis*
35. _____ Both ectocervical and endocervical cells
36. _____ Candidiasis
37. _____ Ectocervical cells

Instrument

a. Dacron swab
b. Wet mount with KOH
c. Spatula
d. Sterile cotton swab
e. Cytobrush
f. Wet mount with NaCl
g. Cervix brush

Copyright © 2003, Mosby, Inc. All rights reserved.

CONCEPTS APPLICATION

Compare and contrast various alternative positions for pelvic examination with the traditional lithotomy pelvic examination position by describing each position below and listing advantages or disadvantages of each.

Position	Description	Advantages/Disadvantages
Knee-chest		
Diamond-shape		
Obstetric stirrups		
M-Shape		
V-Shape		

CASE STUDY

Melinda is a 33-year-old female who presents to the urgent care center. Listed below are data collected by the examiner during the interview and examination.

Interview Data

Melinda tells the examiner, "I have a really bad pain in front of my butt. It hurts so much that I can't even wipe with a tissue after I go to the bathroom." Melinda indicates that the pain started two days ago and is much worse now. When asked about her sexual activity, she says, "I have a guy that I'm with, but it's not exclusive or anything. We see other people and try not to be real serious."

Examination Data

External: Typical hair distribution; urethral meatus intact; no redness or discharge. Perineum intact. Extreme pain response to palpation of vaginal opening. Swelling, redness, and mass detected on right side. Foul-smelling discharge noted.

Internal: Examination deferred because of extreme pain associated with inflammation.

Copyright © 2003, Mosby, Inc. All rights reserved.

1. What data deviate from normal findings, suggesting a need for further investigation?

2. What additional questions could the examiner ask to clarify symptoms?

3. What additional physical examination, if any, should the examiner complete?

4. What primary problems does the patient have?

CRITICAL THINKING

1. Lillian is a 42-year-old blind patient who requests a routine examination. How should the examiner approach this patient to best meet her needs?

2. Judy is a 16-year-old girl who is in the clinic for a school sports physical. How should her health history and an examination of her genitalia differ from that of an adult?

Copyright © 2003, Mosby, Inc. All rights reserved.

18

Male Genitalia

LEARNING OBJECTIVES

After studying Chapter 18 in the textbook and completing this section of the workbook, students should be able to:

1. Conduct a history related to the male genitalia.
2. Discuss examination techniques for the male genitalia.
3. Identify normal age and condition variations of the male genitalia.
4. Recognize findings that deviate from expected findings.
5. Relate symptoms or clinical findings to common pathologic conditions.

TEXTBOOK REVIEW

Chapter 18   Male Genitalia (pages 648–673)

CONTENT REVIEW QUESTIONS

Multiple Choice

Circle the correct answer for each of the following questions.

1. While examining a newborn male infant, the examiner palpates a testicle in the inguinal canal that cannot be pushed into the scrotum. This finding is consistent with:
   a. hydrocele.
   b. ambiguous genitalia.
   c. direct inguinal hernia.
   d. undescended testicle.

2. The examiner is providing a 20-year-old male with information on genital self-examination (GSE). For what reason should a man this age be taught how to do this?
   a. Testicular cancer is the most common type of cancer in young men.
   b. Self-examination can help determine when full development of the genitalia is completed.
   c. Self-examination can prevent acquiring a sexually transmitted disease.
   d. Routine examination can help detect prostate enlargement.

3. The examiner has given a 20-year-old male information regarding GSE. Which statement made by the patient indicates further teaching is necessary?
   a. "I should perform this every month on a regular schedule."
   b. "I should look for discharge or sores on my penis."
   c. "I should look for a hernia while doing this."
   d. "A good time to do this is while bathing."

4. While examining the genitalia of a 2-year-old boy, the examiner should be aware that the:
   a. scrotum is normally edematous.
   b. foreskin of the uncircumcised penis is not fully retractable until age 3 or 4.
   c. testicles typically do not descend into the scrotum until age 5.
   d. supine position is preferred for examination of children this age.

5. Which data collected from the patient history is considered a risk factor for cancer of the penis?
   a. circumcised at birth
   b. history of condyloma acuminatum infections
   c. had a congenital hydrocele
   d. history of untreated epispadias

6. In which of the following situations is transillumination of the scrotum indicated?
   a. Presence of syphilis chancre is noted.
   b. Indirect hernia is palpated.
   c. The examiner suspects a mass.
   d. The examiner palpates the testes.

7. The patient is asked to bear down while the examiner palpates the inguinal ring. The examiner feels a soft swelling sensation on the fingertip. The patient complains of pain while straining. These findings are consistent with which of the following?
   a. indirect hernia
   b. direct hernia
   c. femoral hernia
   d. rectal hernia

8. The examiner inspects the scrotum of a 43-year-old man. Which finding requires further evaluation or follow-up? The:
   a. left testicle hangs lower than the right testicle.
   b. scrotum is darker than the general skin color.
   c. skin on the scrotum is shiny and smooth.
   d. scrotum is divided into two sacs by a septum.

9. Which finding may indicate diabetes?
   a. The vas deferens feels beaded or lumpy.
   b. The testicle feels hard with a lump.
   c. Sebaceous cysts are present on the scrotal skin.
   d. The urethra has a slit-like orifice.

Copyright © 2003, Mosby, Inc. All rights reserved.

10. During an examination for a hernia, an adult male patient should:
    a. be asked to stand.
    b. be in a supine position.
    c. sit on a table with heels together.
    d. assume a knee-chest position on the exam table.

11. Balanitis associated with phimosis occurs only in:
    a. newborn male infants.
    b. diabetic men.
    c. uncircumcised men.
    d. men exposed to radiation.

12. Which of the following testicular characteristics are associated with syphilis or diabetic neuropathy?
    a. asymmetry and dropping
    b. bilateral enlargement
    c. insensitivity to pain
    d. migration into the abdomen

13. What type of hernia would you most likely see with a 15-year-old male?
    a. femoral hernia
    b. umbilical hernia
    c. direct inguinal hernia
    d. indirect inguinal hernia

14. Which of the following scrotal findings is expected for a full-term newborn male?
    a. fibrosis
    b. pendulous
    c. smooth
    d. without rugae

15. A 24-year-old man has scrotal pain and marked erythema. The examiner considers epididymitis. Which finding is consistent with this problem?
    a. An uneven scrotal size and shape is observed.
    b. Patient has anorexia and nausea.
    c. Patient reports an acute onset of severe pain.
    d. Urinalysis shows elevated WBCs and bacteria.

Copyright © 2003, Mosby, Inc. All rights reserved.

Terminology Review

Crossword Puzzle

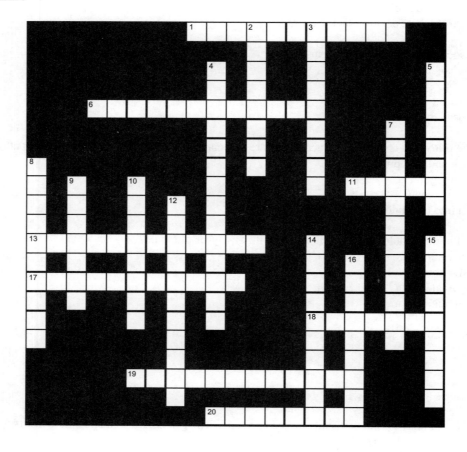

Across

1. A defect on the ventrum of the penis so that the urethral meatus is more proximal than its normal glandular location
6. Inflammation of the epididymis
11. Conical structure at distal aspect of penis
13. Surgical removal of the prepuce
17. Reflex characterized by rising of the scrotum and testicle when the inner thigh is stroked
18. Rotation producing ischemia of testis
19. Cystic swelling on the epididymis
20. Disease characterized by a fibrous band in the corpus cavernosum

Down

2. Acute inflammation of the testis
3. Inflammatory bands that connect opposing serous surfaces
4. Undescended testes
5. Prolonged penile erection
7. Painful constriction of the glans penis by a phimotic foreskin, which has been retracted
8. Abnormal tortuosity and dilation if veins in the spermatic cord
9. Ventral curvature of the penis
10. Narrowness of the opening of the prepuce, preventing its being drawn back over the glans
12. XXY chromosomal anomaly
14. Pattern of hair growth on the male pubis and abdomen
15. Inflammation of the glans
16. Fluid accumulation in the tunica vaginalis resulting in a nontender, smooth, firm mass

Copyright © 2003, Mosby, Inc. All rights reserved.

Matching

Match each lesion descriptor to the corresponding sexually transmitted disease.

Description of Lesion

16. _____ Initially a painless erosion on or near the coronal sulcus
17. _____ Painful superficial vesicles on the glans, penile shaft, or base of the penis
18. _____ Dome-shaped, smooth, pearly gray lesions on the glans penis
19. _____ Painless lesion with clear base and indurated borders, usually located on glans penis
20. _____ Reddish lesions on prepuce, glans, and shaft; may also be present within the urethra

Sexually Transmitted Disease

a. Syphilitic chancre
b. Venereal herpes
c. Genital warts
d. Lymphogranuloma venereum
e. *Molluscum contagiosum*

Match each examination technique to its corresponding purpose.

Examination Technique

21. _____ Foreskin retracted
22. _____ Finger moved along vas deferens
23. _____ Glands pressed between thumb and forefinger
24. _____ Mass transilluminated
25. _____ Testes gently compressed

Purpose

a. Inspecting for urethral discharge
b. Observing for hydrocele
c. Observing for phimosis
d. Palpating for inguinal hernia
e. Palpating for tender testes

CASE STUDY

Mr. Corazza is a 43-year-old male who presents to the urgent care center. Listed below are data collected by the examiner.

Interview Data

Mr. Corazza tells the examiner, "Yesterday I noticed a mild discomfort in my groin. When I looked, I saw this area of swelling." The examiner asks about recent activity. Mr. Corazza replies, "We have been in the process of moving, and I have been picking up heavy boxes, moving furniture, and have been up and down ladders all weekend."

Examination Data

General survey: Healthy-appearing male.

Examination: Bulge noted in area of Hesselbach triangle that is painless. Inguinal area on right side with palpable mass. Pushes against side of finger on examination.

1. What data deviate from normal findings, suggesting a need for further investigation?

Copyright © 2003, Mosby, Inc. All rights reserved.

2. What additional questions could the examiner ask to clarify symptoms?

3. What additional physical examination, if any, should the examiner complete?

4. What primary problems does the patient have?

CRITICAL THINKING

1. A 30-year-old male requests information regarding self-examination of his genitalia. What information should the examiner share with him?

2. When the examiner attempts to examine the genitalia of a 5-year-old boy, the boy refuses to take off his pants and says, "You can't see my privates." What measures can the examiner take to facilitate this part of the exam?

Copyright © 2003, Mosby, Inc. All rights reserved.

Anus, Rectum, and Prostate

LEARNING OBJECTIVES

After studying Chapter 19 in the textbook and completing this section of the workbook, students should be able to:

1. Conduct a history related to the anus, rectum, and prostate.
2. Discuss examination techniques for the anus, rectum, and prostate.
3. Identify normal age and condition variations of the anus, rectum, and prostate.
4. Recognize findings that deviate from expected findings.
5. Relate symptoms or clinical findings to common pathologic conditions.

TEXTBOOK REVIEW

Chapter 19   Anus, Rectum, and Prostate (pages 674–693)

CONTENT REVIEW QUESTIONS

Multiple Choice

Circle the correct answer for each of the following questions.

1. While palpating the lateral and posterior rectal walls, the examiner should expect to palpate:
   a. smooth, even, and uninterrupted surface.
   b. small nodules from internal hemorrhoids.
   c. tissue folds from the valves of Houston.
   d. bulging from the bladder wall.

2. A patient presents with a chief complaint of rectal pain. The examiner will focus the history and examination on which known fact?
   a. Rectal pain is almost always accompanied by an infection.
   b. Rectal pain is almost always an indication of local disease.
   c. A complaint of rectal pain is usually associated with a serious systemic process.
   d. One of the most common causes of rectal pain is prostatic enlargement.

Copyright © 2003, Mosby, Inc. All rights reserved.

3. During an examination, the examiner observes inflammation of the sacrococcygeal area. The patient complains of pain when it is palpated. Which of the following problems is *not* consistent with such a finding?
    a. anorectal fistula
    b. pilonidal cyst
    c. hemorrhoids
    d. perianal abscess

4. While examining the perineum of a 6-year-old girl, the examiner observes hemorrhoids. This finding suggests:
    a. repeated events of sexual abuse.
    b. the presence of chronic constipation.
    c. a diet high in fibrous foods.
    d. an underlying problem such as portal hypertension.

5. To examine a prostate, what surface is palpated?
    a. anterior rectal wall surface
    b. posterior rectal wall surface
    c. anterior prostate surface
    d. deep external sphincter surface

6. A patient tells the examiner she has had clay-colored stools. Stool of this color results from:
    a. a lack of bile pigment.
    b. excessive fiber intake.
    c. excessive dietary beef.
    d. insufficient fluid intake.

7. An elderly male patient is unable to assume a standing position for a routine rectal examination. What is the best alternative position?
    a. lithotomy position
    b. left lateral position with knees flexed
    c. knee-chest position
    d. prone position

8. A pregnant woman presents to the emergency department with the complaint of dark stools. She tells the examiner, "I read in a magazine that this is a sign of bleeding." Which of the following questions by the examiner is most applicable for this situation?
    a. "Where did you read that information?"
    b. "Have you been giving yourself enemas?"
    c. "How much fruit and vegetable intake have you had in the last few days?"
    d. "Are you taking prenatal vitamins?"

9. Prior to palpating the prostate, the examiner should tell the patient that he might feel the urge to do which of the following?
    a. urinate
    b. defecate
    c. vomit
    d. faint

10. Which of the following is considered a routine screening test done in conjunction with a rectal examination?
    a. biopsy of rectal tissue to rule out precancerous cells
    b. smear of rectal lining to rule out infectious disease
    c. transillumination of the rectum to detect a mass
    d. guaiac test of stool to rule out presence of blood

Copyright © 2003, Mosby, Inc. All rights reserved.

11. Which examination finding in the child is a clue to the diagnosis of Hirschsprung's disease?
    a. passing of frequent, loose stools in absence of other symptoms
    b. consistently empty rectum with a history of constipation
    c. itching and irritation around the anus
    d. rectal prolapse

12. In which situation would the examiner perform a rectal examination on an infant or child?
    a. A newborn infant passes a greenish-black viscous stool 12 hours after birth.
    b. The mother of a 3-month-old baby describes the baby's stools as "loose and golden yellow."
    c. A stool of a 6-year-old child is guaiac-positive.
    d. A mother tells the examiner that her 3-year-old child was sent home from day care after two episodes of diarrhea.

13. How is the anal ring assessed?
    a. inspection of the anus
    b. external palpation of the anus
    c. examination of the stool
    d. rotation of a finger within the anal sphincter

14. Which of the following best describes the feel of a normal prostate gland?
    a. soft olive or grape
    b. small sea sponge
    c. Ping-Pong ball
    d. pencil eraser

15. Anal patency is verified in a newborn infant by:
    a. inserting a lubricated thermometer through the anus and into the rectum.
    b. inserting the fifth digit through the anus and into the rectum.
    c. assessing for the passage of a meconium stool in the first 24–48 hours after birth.
    d. inspecting the anus for an anal opening.

16. Prostate enlargement is determined by the:
    a. diameter of the rectum near the bladder.
    b. circumference of the prostate.
    c. estimation of the depth of the sulcus.
    d. protrusion of the prostate into the rectum.

17. Which of the following patients has a known risk factor for colorectal cancer?
    a. Marcus, a 21-year-old college student who is a vegetarian
    b. Jack, a 56-year-old man who eats a diet high in beef
    c. Susan, a 38-year-old with a 5-year history of gastric ulcers
    d. Helen, a 22-year-old mother with multiple hemorrhoids

18. A mother tells the examiner that her 2-year-old son has an odd, bright red bulge coming out of his anus that "looks like a donut." What kind of problem does this history suggest?
    a. pin worms
    b. pilonidal cyst
    c. rectal prolapse
    d. hypertrophy of the anus

19. The examiner palpates a prostate, noting that it is hard and irregular. The median sulcus is not palpable. These findings are consistent with:
    a. prostate cancer.
    b. benign prostate hypertrophy.
    c. prostatitis.
    d. rectal mass.

Copyright © 2003, Mosby, Inc. All rights reserved.

20. A rectal prolapse in a young child is frequently associated with:
    a. rickets.
    b. cystic fibrosis.
    c. Crohn's disease.
    d. chronic constipation or diarrhea.

Terminology Review

Matching

Match each examination finding or symptom to the corresponding problem to be considered.

Examination/Finding/Symptom	Problem
21. _____ Severe rectal pain with a fever	a. Prostatitis
22. _____ Absence of meconium stool passage in infant	b. Perianal abscess
23. _____ Feels smooth and firm with 4 cm protrusion into the rectum	c. Rectal polyp
24. _____ Elevated red granular tissue opening on perianal skin with purulent drainage	d. Benign prostatic hypertrophy
	e. Prostatic carcinoma
25. _____ Feels boggy, enlarged, and tender to palpation	f. Imperforate anus
26. _____ Feels hard, nodular; unable to palpate sulcus	g. Anorectal fistula
27. _____ Soft nodules palpated with rectal examination	

CONCEPTS APPLICATION

Fill in the following table by comparing the different methods for screening prostate cancer.

Screening Method	What It Reflects	What Results Mean	When It Is Indicated
DRE			
PSA			
PSA velocity			
Free PSA ratio			
Biopsy			
TRUS			

Copyright © 2003, Mosby, Inc. All rights reserved.

CASE STUDY

Mr. Murphy is a 66-year-old male who presents to his primary care provider complaining of a 3-month history of rectal fullness. Listed below is data collected by the examiner during an interview and examination.

Interview Data

Mr. Murphy tells the examiner he has had pain "off and on" but became concerned when he started seeing blood in his stool. The blood is described as "bright red." Mr. Murphy also states that he has seen spots on his underwear, but he has ignored it, thinking he had hemorrhoids. When asked about changes in his diet, Mr. Murphy indicates that he really hasn't been very hungry lately and has lost 10 pounds over the last several months.

Examination Data

General survey: Thin-appearing male. Vital signs are within normal limits.

Rectal examination: Perineal and anal inspection is unremarkable with no lesions, dimpling or changes in skin characteristics. Sphincter tone findings unremarkable. A large mass is felt with rectal palpation extending from the posterior to the left lateral rectal wall. The prostate is smooth, firm, and nontender to palpation with a 1 cm protrusion.

1.   What data deviate from normal findings, suggesting a need for further investigation?

2.   What additional questions could the examiner ask to clarify symptoms?

3.   What additional physical examination, if any, should the examiner complete?

4.   What primary problems does the patient have?

Copyright © 2003, Mosby, Inc. All rights reserved.

CRITICAL THINKING

1. A 68-year-old man comes to the emergency department with a history of urinary retention. He states, "I know my bladder is full, but I can't seem to pee." This symptom could be caused by prostatitis, benign prostate hypertrophy, or prostatic carcinoma. How does the examiner differentiate the cause of this patient's symptom?

2. A 70-year-old woman comes to a clinic with a complaint of rectal bleeding. There are multiple causes of rectal bleeding. What kind of interview questions should be asked to help the examiner narrow down the cause of the problem?

Copyright © 2003, Mosby, Inc. All rights reserved.

Musculoskeletal System

LEARNING OBJECTIVES

After studying Chapter 20 in the textbook and completing this section of the workbook, students should be able to:

1. Conduct a history related to the musculoskeletal system.
2. Discuss examination techniques for the musculoskeletal system.
3. Identify normal age and condition variations of the musculoskeletal system.
4. Recognize findings that deviate from expected findings.
5. Relate symptoms or clinical findings to common pathologic conditions.

TEXTBOOK REVIEW

Chapter 20   Musculoskeletal System (pages 694–765)

CONTENT REVIEW QUESTIONS

Multiple Choice

Circle the correct answer for each of the following questions.

1. While examining range of motion (ROM) on a patient, the examiner should remember that:
   a. reverse tailor position is encouraged in adults with limited ROM to the hip.
   b. active ROM is used to assess extremities with complete paralysis.
   c. full muscle strength can be maintained with up to 75% of ROM to the related joint.
   d. passive ROM is normally 5 degrees greater than active ROM.

2. The spine of a newborn infant should be palpated with the examiner noting the shape of each spinal process. If a split is noted in one of the spinal processes, which problem is suspected?
   a. bifid defect
   b. lordosis
   c. Down syndrome
   d. spina bifida

Copyright © 2003, Mosby, Inc. All rights reserved.

3. The examiner observes a 6-month-old infant. Which of the following observations should be considered an expected finding at this age? The infant:
   a. walks around the room holding onto objects.
   b. feeds self with cup and spoon.
   c. holds a rattle or spoon.
   d. sits without support.

4. Which of the following questions asked by the examiner would be most helpful in understanding a patient complaining of acute back pain?
   a. "What medications do you currently take?"
   b. "Was there any activity or injury that occurred prior to the onset of the pain?"
   c. "Were you born with any congenital deformities of the spine?"
   d. "Have you recently lost weight?"

5. Which spinal finding would be considered normal for a 72-year-old patient?
   a. meningocele
   b. myelomeningocele
   c. kyphosis
   d. scoliosis

6. Which of the following data from a patient's history indicates an increased risk of osteomyelitis?
   a. severe gout
   b. rheumatoid arthritis
   c. severe osteoporosis
   d. open fracture of the radius

7. What degree of knee flexion is considered a normal finding?
   a. 15
   b. 90
   c. 130
   d. 160

8. Which of the following is considered a normal finding for a woman in her eighth month of pregnancy?
   a. stronger ligaments and spinal joints
   b. hypercalcemia
   c. 25% loss of muscle strength
   d. lordosis

9. Which of the following conditions would be considered rare among black women?
   a. rheumatoid arthritis
   b. severe osteoporosis
   c. contractures
   d. lordosis

10. When assessing for carpal tunnel syndrome, Tinel's sign can be performed by tapping the:
    a. dorsal aspect of the wrist.
    b. volar carpal ligament.
    c. radial artery.
    d. median nerve.

11. Which group is susceptible to subluxation of the head of the radius?
    a. infants/toddlers
    b. adolescents
    c. pregnant women
    d. older adults

Copyright © 2003, Mosby, Inc. All rights reserved.

12. The extension of the patient's head against the examiner's hand is a test of:
    a. cervical spine alignment.
    b. passive ROM.
    c. temporalis muscle strength.
    d. sternocleidomastoid muscle strength.

13. A patient complains of pain and a clicking noise with jaw movement. The pain extends into the face. These symptoms are suggestive of what condition?
    a. gout in the jaw
    b. temporomandibular joint syndrome
    c. rheumatoid arthritis of the jaw
    d. bursitis of the temporomandibular joint

14. "Normal" muscle strength is documented as Grade _____.
    a. 0
    b. 1
    c. 5
    d. 10

15. While measuring the circumference of extremities of a 43-year-old patient, the examiner makes comparisons of the right and left sides. What findings should the examiner expect?
    a. Measurements between right and left sides should be identical.
    b. Measurement differences are nearly equal.
    c. Measurement differences are within 2 inches.
    d. All of the muscle groups are significantly larger on the dominant side.

16. Which of the following may be an early and subtle symptom of rheumatic fever?
    a. joint pain occurring 10-14 days after a sore throat
    b. swelling and inflammation of joints after exercise
    c. muscle weakness following a fever
    d. reduced ROM in joints occurring 2 weeks after a viral infection

17. To assess muscle strength of the temporalis and masseter muscles, the examiner will ask the patient to:
    a. push the jaw forward while the examiner applies counterforce.
    b. attempt to open his or her mouth while the examiner applies counterforce.
    c. clench his or her teeth while the examiner palpates the contracted muscles.
    d. clench his or her teeth together while the examiner attempts to open the mouth with a tongue blade.

18. For which type of problem does a family history have significance?
    a. rheumatoid arthritis
    b. dislocation of radius
    c. lumbosacral radiculopathy
    d. bursitis

19. The examiner sees two 9-month-old babies on the same day. Jeremy is a black 9 1/2-month-old who pulls himself to a standing position and holds onto a chair while standing. Nathan is a white 9 1/2-month-old who sits alone on the floor using hands for support; his mother states he is not yet scooting or creeping on the floor. What conclusion is appropriate for the examiner to make?
    a. Jeremy is advanced for his age.
    b. Nathan may have a developmental delay.
    c. Jeremy has superior intelligence to Nathan.
    d. Both findings are "normal," considering that Jeremy is black and Nathan is white.

Copyright © 2003, Mosby, Inc. All rights reserved.

20. Which statement made by a patient helps the examiner differentiate osteoarthritis from rheumatoid arthritis? "I:
    a. have swelling and pain in my joints."
    b. notice a crackling sound when I move my joints."
    c. get extremely tired by mid-morning, even when I sleep well."
    d. used to play the piano when I was younger."

Terminology Review

Crossword Puzzle

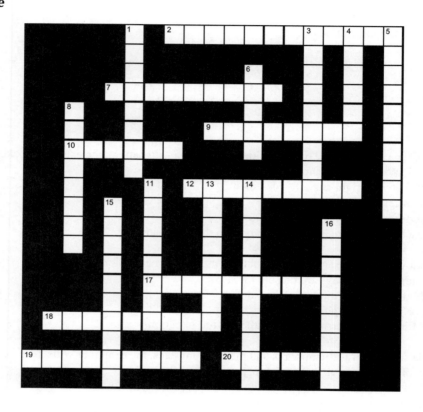

Across

2. Lateral deviation of the great toe with overlapping of the second toe
7. Movement of the extremities toward the body
9. Crackling sound is heard in the patient's joint with movement
10. Single crease extending across the entire palm, associated with Down Syndrome
12. "Flat foot"
17. Position of the forearm when the palm faces upward
18. Movement of the sole of the foot inward at the ankle
19. Flexion deformity at the distal interphalangeal joint of the foot
20. Hyperextension of the metatarsophalangeal joint with flexion of the toe's proximal and distal joints

Down

1. Concave curvature of the lumbar spine
3. Movement of the extremities away from the body
4. Sharp angular deformity associated with a collapsed vertebra from osteoporosis
5. Congenital fusion of digits
6. Sign in children indicating generalized muscle weakness
8. High arch on the sole of the foot
11. Outward curvature of the thoracic spine
13. Movement of the sole of the foot outward at the ankle
14. Presence of more than five digits on hand or foot
15. Calibrated device designed to measure the arc or range of motion of a joint
16. Rotation of the arm so that the palm faces down

Copyright © 2003, Mosby, Inc. All rights reserved.

Matching

Match each examination technique to the problem or condition it is used to detect. Some answers may be used more than once.

Examination Technique

21. _____ Allis' sign
22. _____ Apley test
23. _____ Ballottement
24. _____ Barlow-Ortolani maneuver
25. _____ Bulge sign
26. _____ Drawer test
27. _____ Femoral stretch test
28. _____ Lachman test
29. _____ McMurray test
30. _____ Thomas test
31. _____ Vargus/valgus stress test

Possible Problem/Condition

a. Anterior cruciate ligament injury
b. Effusion of fluid in the knee
c. Flexion contractures in the hip
d. L1, L2, L3, L4 nerve root irritation
e. Torn meniscus in knee
f. Anteroposterior instability in knee
g. Mediolateral instability of knee
h. Hip dislocation

CONCEPTS APPLICATION

Activity 1

Based on the symptoms and/or examination findings provided, list the corresponding problem to consider.

Symptoms/Examination Findings	Problem to Consider
Heberden's nodes and Bouchard's nodes noted on hands	
Low back pain that radiates to the buttocks and posterior thigh, with tenderness over the spine	
Heat, redness, swelling, and tenderness to the metatarsophalangeal joint of the great toe	
Subcutaneous nodules on the forearm near the elbow	
Tenderness, swelling, and boggy sensation with palpation along the grooves of the olecranon process; increased pain with pronation and supination	

Continued next page

Copyright © 2003, Mosby, Inc. All rights reserved.

Symptoms/Examination Findings	Problem to Consider
A child with muscle atrophy and symptoms of progressive muscle weakness	
A child complaining of pain in the elbow and wrist; will not move his or her arm; maintains arm in a flexed and pronated position	

Activity 2

For each developmental task described in the following table, identify the expected age and indicate whether each is a fine motor task or a gross motor task.

Developmental Task	Expected Age	Gross/Fine Motor
Holds crayon; scribbles spontaneously		
Sits with shaky posture; uses tripod position; raises abdomen off table when prone.		
When supine, puts hands together; holds hands in front of face		
Builds a four-block tower; dumps a raisin from a bottle		
Walks alone well; sits self in chair		
Rolls from prone to side position; slight head lag when pulled to sitting position		
Hops on one foot; catches bounced ball; walks heel-to-toe		
Reaches and picks up an object; plays with toes		
Points with one finger		
Begins creeping; stands, holding on, when placed in position		

Copyright © 2003, Mosby, Inc. All rights reserved.

CASE STUDY

Mrs. Simmons is a 46-year-old female with rheumatoid arthritis (RA). Listed below are data collected by the examiner during an interview and examination.

Interview Data

According to the medical record, Mrs. Simmons was diagnosed with RA at the age of 30. Mrs. Simmons complains of a great deal of pain in her joints, particularly in her hands, and says she has just learned to live with the pain because it will always be there. She states that the stiffness and pain in her joints is always worst in the morning, or if she sits around too much. She denies muscle weakness other than the fact that her stiffness and soreness prevent her from doing much. Mrs. Simmons states that the RA is progressing to the point where she is having difficulty doing things requiring fine motor dexterity such as changing clothes, holding utensils to eat, and cutting up her food. She says she can still get cleaned up but had to have different faucet handles placed in her home so that she could turn the water on and off. Mrs. Simmons says she rarely goes out because she feels ugly.

Examination Data

Patient is able to stand, but standing up straight and erect is not possible. Gait is slow and purposeful, with jerky movements. Significant inflammation, swelling, and tenderness is noted with inspection and palpation at hip, knee, wrists, hands, and feet bilaterally. Subcutaneous nodules are noted at ulnar surface of elbows bilaterally.

1. What data deviate from normal findings, suggesting a need for further investigation?

2. What additional questions could the examiner ask to clarify symptoms?

3. What additional physical examination, if any, should the examiner complete?

4. What primary problems does the patient have?

Copyright © 2003, Mosby, Inc. All rights reserved.

CRITICAL THINKING

1. Mark is a 17-year-old who presents with pain to the ankle. He says he twisted it during his soccer game earlier in the afternoon, and now the pain seems to be getting worse. The ankle is very swollen with a bluish discoloration. How does the examiner determine whether Mark has a muscle strain, a sprain, or a fracture?

2. A 2-year-old girl with a dislocation of the radial head is brought to the clinic by her parents. What type of activities could cause such an injury, and what type of teaching should be provided to the parents?

Copyright © 2003, Mosby, Inc. All rights reserved.

21

Neurologic System

LEARNING OBJECTIVES

After studying Chapter 21 in the textbook and completing this section of the workbook, students should be able to:

1. Conduct a history related to the neurologic system.
2. Discuss examination techniques for the neurologic system.
3. Identify normal age and condition variations of the neurologic system.
4. Recognize findings that deviate from expected findings.
5. Relate symptoms or clinical findings to common pathologic conditions.

TEXTBOOK REVIEW

Chapter 21   Neurologic System (pages 766–816)

CONTENT REVIEW QUESTIONS

Multiple Choice

Circle the correct answer for each of the following questions.

1. Which of the following disorders is known to be hereditary?
   a. Creutzfeldt-Jakob disease
   b. meningitis
   c. Huntington's chorea
   d. seizure disorder

2. Unless a problem is suspected, which cranial nerve is not routinely tested?
   a. I
   b. II
   c. V
   d. XI

Copyright © 2003, Mosby, Inc. All rights reserved.

3. The patient is able to rapidly touch each finger to his thumb in rapid sequence. What does this finding mean? The patient has:
   a. intact trochlear and abducens cranial nerves.
   b. appropriate cerebellar function.
   c. an intact spinal accessory nerve.
   d. appropriate kinesthetic sensation.

4. Which question asked by the examiner may help to determine prevention strategies for seizures that a patient is experiencing?
   a. "Where do your seizures typically begin?"
   b. "How do you feel after the seizure?"
   c. "What goes through your mind during the seizure?"
   d. "Are there any factors or activities that seem to start the seizures?"

5. The patient makes the following statement: "I sometimes feel as if the whole room is spinning." What type of neurologic dysfunction should the examiner suspect?
   a. peripheral neuropathy dysfunction
   b. increased intracranial pressure from a brain tumor
   c. inner ear dysfunction affecting the acoustic nerve
   d. lesion affecting the frontal lobe

6. The examiner asks the patient to close her eyes, then places a vibrating tuning fork on the patient's ankle and asks her to indicate what is felt. What is being assessed?
   a. peripheral nerve sensory function
   b. cranial nerve sensory function
   c. cortical sensory function
   d. level of consciousness

7. Which of the following findings should an examiner consider a normal finding if associated with pregnancy?
   a. decreased gag reflex
   b. mild seizures
   c. change in balance
   d. 4+ deep tendon reflexes

8. Sensory neurologic testing is not usually done with children until they are:
   a. preschool age.
   b. kindergarten age.
   c. middle school age.
   d. high school age.

9. Jack is a 52-year-old obese man with a history of poorly controlled diabetes. He also smokes. Based on this data, the examiner should recognize that Jack has several risk factors for:
   a. seizures.
   b. cerebral vascular accident.
   c. multiple sclerosis.
   d. Guillain-Barré syndrome.

Copyright © 2003, Mosby, Inc. All rights reserved.

10. Which of the following assessment findings should not be surprising to an examiner given Jack's history as described in question 9?
    a. inability to discern superficial touch or two-point discrimination on the legs
    b. reduced muscle tone on left side of face
    c. asymmetry of the face when asked to smile and puff out his cheeks
    d. slow and uncoordinated movement with finger-nose test

11. A woman complains of weakness in the lower extremities. She is 2 days postpartum. Which of the following problems should the examiner consider?
    a. depression
    b. obstetric palsy
    c. encephalitis
    d. postpartum stroke

12. The examiner is assessing deep tendon reflex response on a 12-year-old boy. The response is an expected reflex response. Which of the following scores should be documented?
    a. 1+
    b. 2+
    c. 3+
    d. 4+

13. An older patient tells the examiner, "I have a hard time finding the right words when I am talking." This symptom may be:
    a. a precursor to a seizure disorder.
    b. an early symptom of Parkinson's disease.
    c. an indication of a dysfunction of the temporal lobe.
    d. associated with a problem of the vestibular apparatus.

14. What response should occur when a patient's field of gaze moves from a distant object to one close to his or her face?
    a. rapid eye movement
    b. ptosis of the eye
    c. constriction of the pupil
    d. dilation of the iris

15. How can an examiner best gain the cooperation of a child to perform a neurologic examination?
    a. Ask a parent to perform the exam while the examiner observes the response.
    b. Ask the mother or father to step out of the room.
    c. Promise the child a toy or treat if they do what you ask.
    d. Make various aspects of the neurologic examination a game.

16. Which of the following infant reflex responses is considered normal?
    a. A 13-month-old baby's toes fan in response to stroking the lateral surface of the infant's sole.
    b. An 8-month-old infant demonstrates a positive Moro reflex when startled.
    c. A 3-month-old infant's fingers fan when the examiner's finger is placed in the infant's hand.
    d. A 2-month-old infant's legs flex up against the body when the infant is held in an upright position, and the dorsal side of the foot touches the table.

Copyright © 2003, Mosby, Inc. All rights reserved.

17. The examiner is conducting an interview with the mother of an infant as part of the neurologic system examination. Which of the following responses made by the mother may indicate a need for further evaluation?
    a. "My baby sometimes falls asleep when I am feeding her."
    b. "My baby seems to jump when there is a loud noise in the room."
    c. "I drank a glass of wine about once a week while I was pregnant."
    d. "I had problems with hypertension the entire time I was pregnant."

18. A patient demonstrates impaired pain sensation. Which additional test is appropriate to further evaluate this finding?
    a. heat and cold sensation
    b. ultrasonic perception
    c. deep tendon reflex
    d. transillumination of the involved area

19. The examiner squeezes the patient's bicep muscle as part of an examination. Which of the following responses verbalized by the patient is considered normal?
    a. "That makes my arm tingle."
    b. "That makes a burning sensation go up my arm."
    c. "That is uncomfortable."
    d. "My arm is twitching."

20. Which of the following findings is associated with an increased risk of skin breakdown and injury?
    a. inability to feel pressure applied by a monofilament
    b. inability to identify a familiar object by touch
    c. inability to identify a letter drawn in the palm of the hand
    d. 3+ deep tendon reflexes

Copyright © 2003, Mosby, Inc. All rights reserved.

Terminology Review

Crossword Puzzle

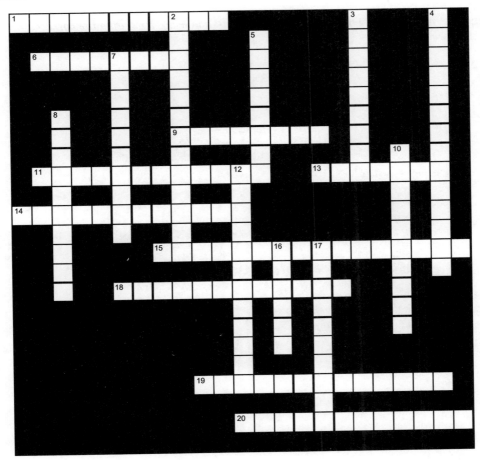

Across

1. Contains the motor cortex; associated with voluntary skeletal movement
6. Behavior used to limit pain, as limping reduces the time of weight bearing on an affected leg
9. Conveys sensory impulses to and from the cerebrum and integrates the impulses between the motor cortex and the cerebrum
11. Responsible for perception and interpretation of sounds, taste, smell, and balance
13. Patient standing with eyes closed is unable to maintain balance when pushed slightly
14. Ability to identify an object by touch
15. Acts as the respiratory center and relay center for major ascending and descending spinal tracts
18. Maintains temperature control, water metabolism, and neuro-endocrine activity
19. Tactual ability to recognize writing on the skin
20. Mediates primitive behaviors that determine survival

Down

2. Contains the primary visual center and interpretation of visual data
3. Acts as the pathway between the cerebral cortex and spinal cord
4. Stiff neck; associated with meningitis
5. Unexpected gait pattern manifested by an excessive lift of the hip and knee and an inability to walk on the heels
7. Absence of deep tendon reflexes may be an indication of this type of neuron disorder or of peripheral neuropathy
8. Works with the motor cortex of the cerebrum; involved in voluntary movement; processes information from eyes, ears, and touch
10. Attempt to straighten a leg of a supine patient with leg flexion at the knee and hip
12. Pathway and processing station between the cerebral motor cortex and the upper brain stem
16. Inability to coordinate muscle activity during voluntary movement
17. Sign characterized by involuntary flexion of the hips and knees when the neck is flexed

Copyright © 2003, Mosby, Inc. All rights reserved.

Anatomy Review

Activity 1

On the following illustration, identify the structures of the skull and brain by writing the correct term in the corresponding lettered answer space.

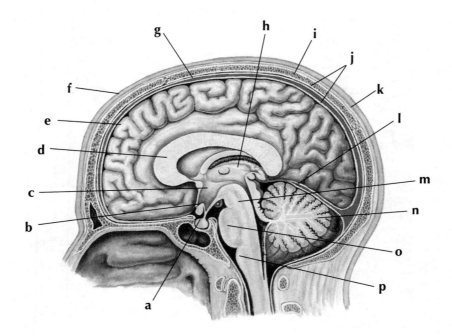

cerebellum
cerebrum
corpus callosum
dura mater (two layers)
galea aponeurotica
hypothalamus
medulla oblongata
midbrain

optic chiasma
pituitary gland
pons
skin
skull
superior sagittal sinus
tentorium cerebelli
thalamus

a. _____

b. _____

c. _____

d. _____

e. _____

f. _____

g. _____

h. _____

i. _____

j. _____

k. _____

l. _____

m. _____

n. _____

o. _____

p. _____

Copyright © 2003, Mosby, Inc. All rights reserved.

Activity 2

On the following illustration, identify the structures of the skull and brain by writing the correct term in the corresponding lettered answer space.

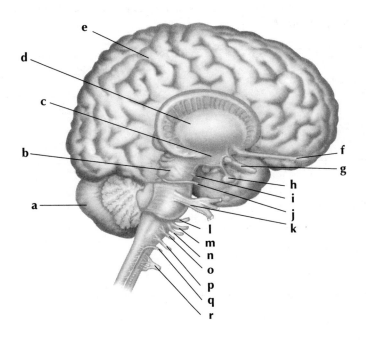

abducens (VI)
acoustic (VIII)
cerebellum
cerebral peduncle
cerebrum
facial (VII)
glossopharyngeal (IX)
hypoglossal (XII)
hypothalamus

oculomotor (III)
olfactory (I)
optic (II)
pituitary gland
spinal accessory (XI)
thalamus
trigeminal (IV)
trochlear (IV)
vagus (X)

a. _____

b. _____

c. _____

d. _____

e. _____

f. _____

g. _____

h. _____

i. _____

j. _____

k. _____

l. _____

m. _____

n. _____

o. _____

p. _____

q. _____

r. _____

Copyright © 2003, Mosby, Inc. All rights reserved.

CONCEPTS APPLICATION

Activity 1

Complete the following table by writing in the cranial nerve(s) tested by each examination procedure. More than one cranial nerve may be tested with each procedure.

Examination Procedure	*Cranial Nerve Tested*
Whisper test	
Patient sticking out tongue and moving it from side to side	
Taste test with sugar, salt, and lemon	
Visual acuity	
Patient puffing out cheeks and showing teeth	
Patient shrugging shoulders against examiner's hands	
Smell test with coffee, orange, and cloves	
Eyes constricting and dilating in response to light	
Patient clenching teeth (temporal muscles contracted)	

Copyright © 2003, Mosby, Inc. All rights reserved.

Activity 2

In the table below, write the name of the reflex based on the observed response; then indicate whether this is expected or unexpected, based on the age of the infant and/or the nature of the response.

Age of Infant	Observed Response	Name of Reflex	Expected/Unexpected
8 months	The infant abducts and extends arms and legs in response to sudden movement of head and trunk backward. The arms then adduct in an embracing motion followed by relaxation.		
2 months	The infant demonstrates a strong grasp of the examiner's finger when it is placed in the infant's palm.		
4 months	When held in an upright position with soles of the feet touching the surface of a table, the infant flexes legs upward in a curled position and holds them there.		
6 months	In a suspended head-first prone position, the infant extends arms and legs.		

CASE STUDY

Melvin Thomas is a 64-year-old male admitted to the hospital with a diagnosis of acute cerebral vascular accident (CVA). Listed below are data collected by the examiner during an interview and examination.

Interview Data

Mr. Thomas's wife tells the examiner that her husband was fine until this morning when he suddenly had a headache, fell to the floor, and could not get up. Mrs. Thomas adds that when she tried to get her husband to speak, he made only mumbling noises, and she could not understand him.

Examination Data

Mental status: Awake, alert male. Unable to talk, but able to follow commands. Very distraught over this incident. Patient cries and avoids eye contact with the wife and examiner.

Copyright © 2003, Mosby, Inc. All rights reserved.

Neurologic examination: Cranial nerves I, II, III, IV, V, VI, VIII all intact. Patient has asymmetry and unequal movements of face, with a drooping of the left side of face. Has asymmetry of shoulder shrug, with deficiency noted on left side. Patient has left-sided paralysis. Demonstrates expected muscle tone and sensation on right side. Unable to assess balance. Unable to get up or move around in bed unassisted at this time.

1. What data deviate from normal findings, suggesting a need for further investigation?

2. What additional questions could the examiner ask to clarify symptoms?

3. What additional physical examination, if any, should the examiner complete?

4. What primary problems does the patient have?

CRITICAL THINKING

1. Kevin, an ambitious novice examiner, uses an unfolded paper clip to test peripheral two-point discrimination. He adjusts the paper clip so that the points are 1 inch apart. With this instrument, he tests the patient's palm, toe, back, upper arm, and upper leg, and he notes that the patient fails to discriminate between one and two points in each of these areas. Kevin concludes that the patient has some sort of peripheral sensory deficit. What is incorrect in Kevin's methods and/or conclusion?

2. The CT scan of a patient demonstrates an infarction of the frontal lobe toward the left side. What brain functions occur in the frontal lobe? What type of symptoms would you anticipate this patient to have?

Copyright © 2003, Mosby, Inc. All rights reserved.

22

Putting It All Together

LEARNING OBJECTIVES

After studying Chapter 22 in the textbook and completing this section of the workbook, students should be able to:

1. Discuss the process of completing the history and physical examination.
2. Describe patient reliability and factors that may affect accuracy of data collected.
3. Describe general examination sequence.
4. Identify techniques useful for evaluation of infants and young children.
5. Discuss the functional assessment.

TEXTBOOK REVIEW

Chapter 22   Putting It All Together (pages 817–846)

CONTENT REVIEW QUESTIONS

Multiple Choice

Circle the correct answer for each of the following questions.

1. When performing a physical examination, you should consider the examination to begin:
   a. as soon as you meet the patient.
   b. after the vital signs are taken.
   c. after you explain to the patient everything you are going to do.
   d. after the patient has put on an exam gown.

2. The examiner may decide to omit various aspects of an examination. Which of the following best explains how that decision is made?
   a. The patient is feeling ill.
   b. The patient already knows what is wrong, and a diagnosis can be based on the history.
   c. Certain examination steps will provide data of limited value.
   d. Anxiety is observed by the examiner.

Copyright © 2003, Mosby, Inc. All rights reserved.

3. In what way can the patient's modesty be maintained while an examination is being conducted? The examiner should:
   a. turn his or her back while the patient undresses.
   b. keep the patient covered as much as possible during the examination.
   c. avoid touching the patient during the examination except when absolutely necessary.
   d. not require the patient to disrobe for the examination.

4. Which examination approach is suggested for a 14-month-old baby? The baby should be:
   a. completely undressed and lying down on an examination table.
   b. fully clothed and placed on the floor with toys; the examiner should conduct the examination while the child plays.
   c. completely undressed and held by the examiner.
   d. wearing only a diaper and sitting on his or her parent's lap.

5. Which examination technique is not generally included in the examination of a newborn infant?
   a. percussion of the chest
   b. palpation of the abdomen
   c. auscultation of the lungs
   d. inspection of the mouth and palate

6. Which of the following assists the examiner in determining the gestational age of a newborn infant?
   a. measurement of the head circumference
   b. percussion to determine liver size
   c. inspection of hair distribution of the scalp
   d. inspection of the sole of the foot

7. A patient complains of a sore throat. Which aspect of the examination could be eliminated?
   a. vital signs
   b. palpation of lymph nodes
   c. deep tendon reflexes
   d. auscultation of the heart and lungs

8. All of the following can be assessed initially during the general inspection *except*:
   a. mobility.
   b. nutritional status.
   c. urinary function.
   d. skin color.

9. What technique will most likely facilitate the examination of a small frightened girl?
   a. Promise the child you won't hurt her.
   b. Tell the child a story in order to distract her.
   c. Use restraints to hold the child, but tell her you are playing a game with her.
   d. Tell the child you will give her a toy or treat if she does not cry.

10. Which of the following aspects of examination is most relevant to the evaluation of an older adult?
    a. functional assessment
    b. physical measurements
    c. developmental scoring
    d. vital signs, including peripheral pulse examination

11. For a routine physical examination, all of the following equipment is necessary *except*:
    a. pen light.
    b. measuring tape.
    c. examination gloves.
    d. monofilament.

Copyright © 2003, Mosby, Inc. All rights reserved.

12. Which of the following best describes how the collection of a history should be done? It:
    a. is always done at the very beginning of an examination to help you identify problems.
    b. is done at the end of the physical examination after you have identified problems.
    c. may be done before, during, and after the examination.
    d. is done only if it is relevant to the situation.

Terminology Review

Matching

Mr. Walker is a 62-year-old man requiring a routine physical examination. Below is a list of some of the procedures that will be performed during the examination, as well as some of the equipment that will be needed. Match the type of equipment needed to the corresponding examination procedure. Answers may be used more than once; some procedures require more than one answer.

Examination Procedure	**Equipment Needed**
13. _____ Red reflex	a. Eye chart (Snellen)
14. _____ Lung sounds	b. Gloves
15. _____ Jugular venous pulsations	c. Lubricant
16. _____ Symmetry of muscle groups	d. Marking pen
17. _____ Gag reflex	e. Measuring tape
18. _____ Thyroid	f. Ophthalmoscope
19. _____ Rectal and prostate exam	g. Otoscope
20. _____ Tympanic membrane	h. Penlight
21. _____ Visual acuity	i. Percussion hammer
22. _____ Rinne and Weber tests	j. Stethoscope
23. _____ Liver span	k. Tongue blade
24. _____ Lymph nodes	l. Tuning fork
25. _____ Heart murmurs	m. No equipment needed
26. _____ Deep tendon reflex	
27. _____ Romberg test	
28. _____ Retinal examination	
29. _____ Bowel sounds	
30. _____ Tactile fremitus	

Copyright © 2003, Mosby, Inc. All rights reserved.

CONCEPTS APPLICATION

Activity 1

Complete the following table by listing the body systems examined in each of the examination areas provided in the left column. Select the appropriate body systems from those provided in the box. You will use some systems more than once.

Examination Area	Body Systems Examined
Upper extremities	
Anterior chest	
Abdomen	
Head and neck	

Activity 2

Next to each patient position, list the procedures that should be included during an examination in that position. This information is provided in your textbook, but try to complete this activity as much as possible based on your memory of what you have learned.

Position	Examination Procedures to Be Included

Copyright © 2003, Mosby, Inc. All rights reserved.

Position	*Examination Procedures to Be Included*

Copyright © 2003, Mosby, Inc. All rights reserved.

CRITICAL THINKING

1. A 61-year-old blind female patient presents for a yearly physical examination. What type of modification, if any, should be made to individualize your examination approach and/or procedures for this individual?

2. A 43-year-old man presents for his 6-month physical examination. He has multiple health problems, including diabetes and coronary artery disease. From the onset of the examination, he is overbearing; he begins questioning your techniques and your abilities. He indicates that he is an important person in the community and knows many people of importance. What things can you do to gain this individual's confidence and decrease his anxiety?

Copyright © 2003, Mosby, Inc. All rights reserved.

Taking the Next Steps: Critical Thinking

LEARNING OBJECTIVES

After studying Chapter 23 in the textbook and completing this section of the workbook, students should be able to:

1. Discuss the process of data analysis.
2. Describe barriers to critical thinking in reaching diagnostic conclusions.
3. Identify terms associated with data analysis and problem identification.
4. Discuss the role of additional testing in the clinical examination process.
5. Describe what is meant by *patient management plan*, and explain where it fits with critical thinking and clinical examination.

TEXTBOOK REVIEW

Chapter 23   Taking the Next Steps: Critical Thinking (pages 847-854)

CONTENT REVIEW QUESTIONS

Multiple Choice

Circle the correct answer for each of the following questions.

1. Unless a life-threatening situation exists, the best guide to determining the priority for the patient's condition should be based on:
   a. intuition.
   b. probability and utility.
   c. the use of algorithms.
   d. the examiner's initial favorite hypothesis.

Copyright © 2003, Mosby, Inc. All rights reserved.

2. When determining a need for additional examination, testing, or procedures, one should consider that they should be done:
    a. to obtain as much data as possible.
    b. to attempt to get data that might be associated with multiple problems.
    c. only when it is absolutely necessary.
    d. if they relate to the examiner's hypothesis.

3. After an examiner has identified and confirmed a problem, the next step is to:
    a. assess the data collected.
    b. formulate a clinical opinion.
    c. conduct further assessment.
    d. determine the management plan.

4. The use of a computer could potentially be detrimental to the examiner because:
    a. it may become a substitute for critical thinking.
    b. computer dysfunction makes it unreliable.
    c. the computer is limited in the amount of data it can interpret.
    d. the level of skill needed to run a diagnostic computer program is beyond the computer skills of most examiners.

5. In order to identify problems based on clinical examination, it is helpful to organize the data:
    a. by dividing data into normal and abnormal findings.
    b. by body systems.
    c. by chief complaints.
    d. in the order the data was collected.

6. Each of the following could become a barrier to the critical thinking process *except* for the examiner's:
    a. feelings.
    b. attitudes.
    c. values.
    d. objectivity.

7. Which statement best characterizes a belief that supports a sound decision-making process?
    a. The underlying problem is always related to the chief complaint.
    b. Rare problems tend to have unusual presentations.
    c. Common problems occur commonly, whereas rare ones occur rarely.
    d. A diagnosis should be made quickly to enhance patient confidence.

8. Lab tests should be used to:
    a. confirm a presumed diagnosis.
    b. develop a list of potential problems.
    c. rule out all possible causes of symptoms and clinical findings.
    d. assist the examiner only when the data does not point to a specific problem.

Copyright © 2003, Mosby, Inc. All rights reserved.

Terminology Review

Matching

Match each example with the correct term in the right column. Use each choice only once.

Example	Term
9. _____ The examiner notes a positive Homan's sign in the absence of thrombophlebitis.	a. Bayes' formula
10. _____ Based on observations made, the examiner correctly concludes that a patient does not have renal disease.	b. false negative
11. _____ The patient does not demonstrate tenderness at McBurney's point, and does not have appendicitis.	c. false positive
12. _____ A numeric value is assigned, predicting the probability that a patient with negative findings does not have a given illness or condition.	d. negative predictive value
13. _____ A diagnosis of hepatitis B is made on a patient based on his symptoms and the population of IV drug abusers of which he is part.	e. positive predictive value
14. _____ The examiner correctly concludes that a patient has chronic hypoxia based on the patient's presentation.	f. sensitivity
15. _____ A patient with cholecystitis has a positive Murphy's sign.	g. specificity
16. _____ The examiner notes normal findings on a patient with cancer of the prostate.	h. true positive
17. _____ With acute myocardial infarction, 90% of patients demonstrate diaphoresis.	i. true negative

---

CONCEPTS APPLICATION

Activity 1

Complete the following table by listing the body systems that might be involved with each of the symptoms described. Choose body systems from those listed in the box. All symptoms have more than one possible body system involvement; answers can be used more than once.

Body Systems
auditory   cardiovascular   gastrointestinal   integumentary   musculoskeletal   neurologic   respiratory   visual

Symptoms	Body Systems That Might Be Involved
Chest pain	
Headaches	
Abdominal pain	
Pain in the legs	

Copyright © 2003, Mosby, Inc. All rights reserved.

Activity 2

Complete the following table by listing possible problems associated with the examination data provided.

Examination Data	Possible Problems
54-year-old female with jaundice, abdominal pain, nausea, weight loss. Has pain to abdominal palpation; positive bowel sounds. Liver slightly enlarged; admits to alcohol use.	
66-year-old male with chief complaint of breathing difficulty. Has increased respiratory rate, low-grade fever, rales, productive cough; increased tactile fremitus bilaterally.	
13-week-old infant girl with fever, irritability, poor eating. Infant is dehydrated and has a temperature of 103.7° F; abdomen soft.	
19-year-old female college student with chief complaint of pain when urinating. Describes frequency and urgency. Patient has temperature of 100.4° F; Has constant pain in pelvic area; positive pain with fist percussion over left flank.	

Copyright © 2003, Mosby, Inc. All rights reserved.

Recording Information

LEARNING OBJECTIVES

After studying Chapter 24 in the textbook and completing this section of the workbook, students should be able to:

1. Describe reasons for maintaining clear and accurate records.
2. Discuss various components of the POMR.
3. Organize data in appropriate system sections of the history.
4. Delineate methods for documenting the location and description of findings.

TEXTBOOK REVIEW

Chapter 24   Recording Information (pages 855-884)

CONTENT REVIEW QUESTIONS

Multiple Choice

Circle the correct answer for each of the following questions.

1. Which of the following examples illustrates a vague or nondescriptive term? "Skin:
   a. color is normal."
   b. turgor is elastic."
   c. is thin and smooth."
   d. is warm and dry."

2. How are "normal findings" best documented?
   a. Write *normal* or *within normal limits* on the documentation form.
   b. Write *NA* (not applicable) on the documentation sheet.
   c. Because documentation focuses on abnormal findings, do not write anything down for normal findings.
   d. Document what was actually assessed in specific terms.

Copyright © 2003, Mosby, Inc. All rights reserved.

3. One way that a health history for an infant differs from that of an adult is the inclusion of:
    a. nutritional history.
    b. chief complaint.
    c. prenatal information.
    d. personal social information.

4. If a mistake is made in the patient record, it is suggested that a line be drawn through it so that it is still legible. The basis for this action is related to the fact that:
    a. no errors are allowed.
    b. the chart is a legal document.
    c. a pen is messy when used to obliterate writing.
    d. others may want to read what your first impressions were.

5. Which of the following issues has most recently challenged the health care system regarding privacy of patient records?
    a. inclusion of sensitive details regarding family and social data
    b. access to the record by multiple health care professionals
    c. students in the health care delivery area who do not appropriately handle patient confidentiality
    d. computer-based health data systems

6. A 4-year-old girl has fallen against a coffee table and has knocked out all of her incisors. How is this best documented by the examiner?
    a. Teeth missing: 11, 21, 31, 41
    b. Teeth missing: 51, 61, 71, 81
    c. No teeth: 11, 12, 13, 14
    d. "Knocked out all the incisors"

7. Which of the following statements is true regarding use of abbreviations?
    a. Use of any abbreviations is fine as long as you can interpret them.
    b. Abbreviations should be used as much as possible to reduce time and space needed for documentation.
    c. Abbreviations should be avoided because they are not considered acceptable.
    d. Use only universally accepted abbreviations for documentation.

8. The examiner can substantially reduce the possibility of legal problems by:
    a. maintaining clear medical records.
    b. using SOAP format to document all entries.
    c. using a POMR.
    d. drawing genograms in the patient record.

9. Which of the following information belongs in a family history?
    a. chronic illness
    b. current problems
    c. hereditary diseases
    d. personal data

10. A drawing in the medical record may be used to document:
    a. pulse amplitude.
    b. location of lesions.
    c. location of mass.
    d. all of the above.

Copyright © 2003, Mosby, Inc. All rights reserved.

Terminology Review

Fill in the blanks in the following statements, selecting appropriate terms from the word choice box.

Word Choice Box

Uniform Dental Recording System	subjective	SOAP
illustration	POMR	chief complaint
objective	health history	incremental grading
physical examination		

---

11. _____ data is collected during the history and is based on patient reports.

12. A brief description of the patient's main reason for seeking health care is referred to as the

_____.

13. _____ is a format used to document health history notes.

14. The use of stick people to document findings is an example of using a(n) _____.

15. The _____ is a system used to document location of teeth.

16. _____ data is collected while conducting the physical examination.

17. _____ is the use of recorded numbers to represent findings by variable degrees.

18. The _____ is a widely accepted medical record format.

19. The _____ is the part of the record where information from a patient interview is recorded.

20. Clinical findings are recorded during the _____.

Copyright © 2003, Mosby, Inc. All rights reserved.

CONCEPTS APPLICATION

Develop a problem list for Mrs. Olivas based on the following information:

Mrs. Olivas comes to the clinic complaining of back pain. She indicates this pain started in June 1998, while moving some rocks in her garden. Other pertinent aspects of her history include insulin-dependent diabetes mellitus (IDDM) since 1977, which she says she has never really had under control, and cholecystitis for which she had a cholecystectomy in May 1997. Mrs. Olivas has a family history of atherosclerotic heart disease (ASHD) and chronic renal failure (CRF).

Problem #	*Onset*	*Problem*	*Date Resolved*

Copyright © 2003, Mosby, Inc. All rights reserved.

CASE STUDY

Jean is a 37-year-old female who has been interviewed for a health history. Her family history is given in the following paragraph. In the space below, draw a genogram for Jean's family history using the information provided.

Jean is married. Her husband is 43. The couple have a 12-year-old son, an 11-year-old daughter, and a 10-year-old son, all in good health. Jean has a 42-year-old brother and three sisters aged 40, 36, and 32. All of her siblings are in good health. Both of Jean's parents are alive. Her 70-year-old father has mild emphysema and is an only child. Her mother is 66 and has hypertension. Jean's mother has three siblings; the oldest (Jean's uncle) is 74 and suffers from glaucoma. Another brother is 72 and is in good health. A sister is 69 and has osteoarthritis. All of Jean's grandparents are deceased. Her paternal grandfather died at the age of 89 of prostate cancer. Her paternal grandmother died of congestive heart failure at the age of 91. Jean's maternal grandfather died at the age of 86 of prostate cancer, and her maternal grandmother died of "old age" at the age of 96.

Copyright © 2003, Mosby, Inc. All rights reserved.

CRITICAL THINKING

1. The onset of a "new" symptom should be thoroughly documented. Describe what the mnemonic "OLDCARTS" refers to regarding documentation of a symptom.

    O:

    L:

    D:

    C:

    A:

    R:

    T:

    S:

2. While examining a patient, you note a mass. What characteristics should be described when documenting any organ, mass, or lesion?

Copyright © 2003, Mosby, Inc. All rights reserved.

25

Emergency or
Life-Threatening Situations

LEARNING OBJECTIVES

After studying Chapter 25 in the textbook and completing this section of the workbook, students should be able to:

1. Compare and contrast primary and secondary assessment.
2. Describe findings considered significant in the secondary assessment.
3. Describe how pediatric emergency assessment differs from adult emergency assessment.
4. Identify pediatric findings considered to be of concern or ominous.
5. Discuss the impact of advance directives on providing immediate care.

TEXTBOOK REVIEW

Chapter 25   Emergency or Life-Threatening Situations (pages 885-903)

CONTENT REVIEW QUESTIONS

Multiple Choice

Circle the correct answer for each of the following questions.

1. Approximately how long should an examiner take to conduct a primary assessment of the stable patient?
    a. 30 seconds
    b. 60 seconds
    c. 2 minutes
    d. 5 minutes

2. After the initial primary assessment is conducted, how often should it be repeated?
    a. every 30 seconds
    b. every 2 minutes
    c. every 5 minutes
    d. every time the patient's condition changes

Copyright © 2003, Mosby, Inc. All rights reserved.

3. Which finding is consistent with abdominal hemorrhage?
   a. increased bowel sounds
   b. distention and pain
   c. hyperresonance with percussion
   d. auscultation of mesentery artery

4. Which of the following findings suggests a serious problem in a 3-year-old child who has fallen from a tree?
   a. respiratory rate of 38
   b. pulse rate of 164
   c. lethargy
   d. crying

5. Mike complains of severe rib pain. His coworkers state he was hurt on the job when a large pipe struck him across the chest. Given this history, which type of problem should be considered during the secondary assessment?
   a. flail chest
   b. rebound tenderness
   c. pulmonary embolus
   d. pupillary constriction

6. A patient from a motor vehicle accident presents with a suspected neck injury. Which of the following actions by the examiner is clearly *not* appropriate?
   a. assessing peripheral pulses
   b. providing airway support
   c. logrolling the patient to assess his back
   d. hyperextending the neck to establish an airway

7. With which of the following clinical problems would crepitation be an expected finding?
   a. myocardial infarction
   b. cardiovascular accident
   c. blunt abdominal trauma
   d. pneumothorax

8. During the primary assessment, the examiner asks the patient, "Can you tell me who you are?" This question assesses:
   a. airway and orientation.
   b. exposure and circulation.
   c. breathing and circulation.
   d. disability and exposure.

9. Which of the following findings suggests poor peripheral perfusion?
   a. rapid heart rate
   b. dorsalis pedis pulse with 3+ amplitude
   c. capillary refill > 2 seconds
   d. radial pulse palpable

10. A child is struck by a car while riding his bike. Upon arrival at the hospital, the child is not breathing. Which of the following best describes the appropriate actions of an examiner?
    a. Conduct a primary and secondary assessment before deciding what care to provide.
    b. Conduct a primary assessment; before starting a secondary assessment, support breathing.
    c. Stop the primary assessment as soon as the apnea is recognized in order to perform interventions to stabilize the breathing.
    d. Appropriate action depends on the degree of cyanosis observed by the examiner.

Copyright © 2003, Mosby, Inc. All rights reserved.

11. A patient displays Cushing's triad (a drop in pulse rate, rise in blood pressure, and widened pulse pressure). With which type of life-threatening condition are such clinical findings associated?
    a. myocardial infarction
    b. ruptured cerebral aneurysm
    c. status asthmaticus
    d. status epilepticus

12. An examiner suspects that a patient has a cervical spine injury. The examiner can rule out this possibility by:
    a. examining peripheral motor and sensation.
    b. assessing level of consciousness.
    c. assessing for pain and deformity.
    d. acquiring x-rays of all cervical vertebrae.

13. During primary assessment, the examiner notes dampness inside a trauma victim's dark-colored coat. Which of the following is most important for the examiner to determine as the cause of this dampness?
    a. severe sweating
    b. urine
    c. IV fluids
    d. blood

14. A patient presents with a complaint of a sudden flashes of light in the field of vision. What other symptom commonly accompanies this primary symptom?
    a. severe nausea and vomiting
    b. partial loss of vision
    c. severe pain to the eye
    d. intense dizziness

15. A man is shot and critically wounded in a domestic dispute. From a legal standpoint, the health care providers must:
    a. obtain written consent from the patient prior to providing care.
    b. call the police prior to providing care.
    c. save all items from the patient for law enforcement personnel while providing care.
    d. determine whether the man has advance directives prior to providing care.

Terminology Review

Matching

Match the clinical sign to the condition(s) with which it is likely to be associated. Answers may be used more than once; some conditions have more than one answer.

Condition	**Clinical Sign**
16. _____ Ectopic pregnancy	a. Battle's sign
17. _____ Pneumothorax	b. Cullen's sign
18. _____ Basilar skull fracture	c. Grey-Turner's sign
19. _____ Retroperitoneal hematoma	d. Hamman's crunch
20. _____ Facial fracture	e. Kehr's sign
21. _____ Blunt injury to abdomen	f. Raccoon eyes

Copyright © 2003, Mosby, Inc. All rights reserved.

CONCEPTS APPLICATION

Activity 1

Indicate whether the action described would be part of a primary or secondary assessment in a patient with a life-threatening condition.

1. _____ Removing clothing from a patient with an abdominal gunshot wound

2. _____ Performing a Glasgow Coma Scale

3. _____ Taking a history of injury

4. _____ Stabilizing the cervical spine

5. _____ Auscultating the heart

6. _____ Taking vital signs

7. _____ Managing a large, pulsating, bleeding wound

8. _____ Assessing for presence of breathing

9. _____ Assessing the abdomen for internal bleeding

10. _____ Conducting diagnostic tests

11. _____ Assessing peripheral pulses

CASE STUDY

Mark O'Neil is a 19-year-old male rushed to the emergency room by his roommate.

Primary Assessment

Upon arrival, Mark is extremely anxious with profound dyspnea. He states, "Please help me. I can't breathe enough air—something is wrong with me! My chest hurts all over, and I can't breathe!" The examiner notes a large, muscular, healthy-appearing male in acute respiratory distress. Nasal flaring is noted with cyanosis around the lips. Overall impression is that of hypoxia.

1. Based on this information, list your primary assessment findings:
   A:

   B:

Copyright © 2003, Mosby, Inc. All rights reserved.

C:

D:

E:

2. What type of treatment should be initiated immediately during the primary assessment?

3. What is the first thing that should be assessed at the onset of the secondary assessment?

Secondary Assessment: Subjective Data

Mark's roommate tells you that Mark is very athletic and very healthy. "He plays college football and had surgery on his knee two weeks ago because of an injury this past season. This evening he was fine—we were watching TV. Then when he got up to go into the kitchen, he called for help and told me to get him to the hospital now! All that happened about 20 minutes ago." The roommate states, "Mark does not use any drugs. He drinks beer and stuff, but nothing tonight."

Secondary Assessment: Objective Data

Vital signs: Pulse 142. Respiratory rate 40. Blood pressure 138/84. Temperature 99.1° F.

Skin color: Generally pale with cyanosis around lips and in nail beds.

Head/Neck: Pupils reactive to light. Oral cavity WNL.

Chest: Breath sounds auscultated in all lung fields. Has productive cough with bloody sputum. Heart sounds WNL.

Abdomen: Bowel sounds present. No pain; soft, nondistended.

Extremities: Pulses palpable in all extremities; no swelling.

Neurologic: Awake, but not following all commands; extremely anxious.

Arterial blood gas: pH 7.31; O_2 63; PCO_2 69 (respiratory acidosis).

Copyright © 2003, Mosby, Inc. All rights reserved.

4. What data deviate from normal?

5. What additional secondary assessment would you plan to conduct?

6. Based on the information presented, what problems do you think this patient might be experiencing?

CRITICAL THINKING

1. You are examining a 2-year-old boy with a fever. During your assessment, you note that the child has dry mucous membranes and tenting of skin, although his skin color is pink. His breathing is rapid but unlabored. He wants to be held by his mother and cries off and on in a whimpering fashion. The child avoids eye contact with you; he has a dull affect and fails to smile. Based on the Yale Observation Scales for Children, what score would you give this child? What does this score reflect?

2. Mrs. Martin and her 3-year-old daughter Amanda are brought to the hospital for emergency care after being burned in a house fire.

    a. In addition to the burns, what types of problems should the examiner rule out on both of these patients?

    b. What anatomical differences between Amanda and her mother will affect how they are examined?

Copyright © 2003, Mosby, Inc. All rights reserved.

Answer Key

CHAPTER 1

Content Review Questions

Multiple Choice

1. c
2. c
3. b
4. c
5. d
6. a
7. b
8. b
9. a
10. c
11. c
12. a
13. c
14. d
15. c
16. d
17. b
18. d
19. a
20. d
21. a
22. b

Terminology Review

Matching

23. h
24. d
25. f
26. j

Copyright © 2003, Mosby, Inc. All rights reserved.

27. c
28. e
29. g
30. a
31. i
32. b

Crossword Puzzle

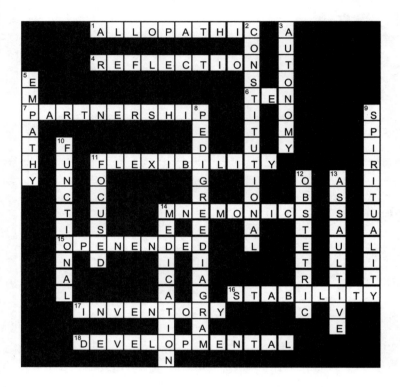

Concepts Application

Activity 1

1. Do a focused history, which would include the following: chief complaint, medical history, allergies, and history regarding the accident, including inquiring about loss of consciousness.
2. Do a complete history. For a pregnancy, this would include chief complaint, age, marital status, occupation, information about the father, obstetric history (including LMP, expected delivery date, gravidity, parity, and use of contraception or contraceptive history), medical history, family history, personal and social history, review of symptoms and risk assessment.
3. Do an interim history, which would include chief complaint and present problem (including a chronicle of events that have occurred since last visit).

Copyright © 2003, Mosby, Inc. All rights reserved.

Activity 2

Patient Behavior	Examiner Behavior to Decrease Tension
Seduction	Do not respond to seductive behavior. Be courteous, calm, firm, and direct from the start; send the message that the relationship is, and will remain, professional.
Dissembling	Do not neglect it. Allow the interview to continue, but come back with gentle questioning to indicate you feel there may be more to the story than what has been discussed.
Anxiety	Avoid overload of information. Pace the conversation with a calm demeanor; avoid allowing the anxiety to become contagious.
Excessive flattery	Be aware that this is possibly a manipulation on the part of the patient; it is easy to be taken in by such manipulations.
Financial concerns	Be aware that the patient may be concerned about the cost of health care; be prepared to talk about it with the patient.

Case Study

Relevant Question	Patient Data You Already Know	Questions You Should Ask
Where?	Lower back pain	Does the pain move to other locations? If so, where?
When?	Pain for 2 days; worse in AM and late at night; comes and goes during the day.	What happened the morning you woke up? What happened the day before the pain started? Does the pain ever subside completely? For how long does it subside?
What?	None	What makes the pain better? What makes the pain worse?
How?	Pain has caused irritability and inability to work.	Does it affect your ability to do personal activities (get dressed, take a shower, make dinner, sit in a chair)?
Why?	None	Why do you think your back may have begun to hurt? What do you think caused this?

Copyright © 2003, Mosby, Inc. All rights reserved.

CHAPTER 2

Content Review Questions

Multiple Choice

1. b
2. d
3. c
4. d
5. a
6. b
7. b
8. c
9. a
10. c
11. b
12. d
13. d
14. a

Terminology Review

15. cultural competency
16. Doing Orientation
17. change
18. *yin* and *yang*
19. primacy

Matching

20. d
21. c
22. j
23. e
24. i
25. h
26. b
27. a
28. g
29. f

Copyright © 2003, Mosby, Inc. All rights reserved.

Crossword Puzzle

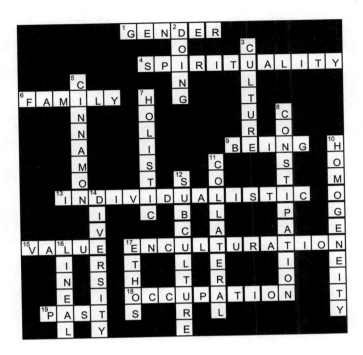

Critical Thinking

1. Ask the mother and/or grandmother about the cloth. Ask permission to remove the cloth long enough to examine the abdomen, with the understanding that it may be placed back on when you are finished.

2. *Health belief and practices*: What does illness mean to you? How do you perceive your health? What do you currently do to treat your illness and to help you stay healthy?

   Religious and ritual influences: Do you have any special religious practices or beliefs? Are there any special practices or beliefs that may affect health care when the patient is ill or dying?

   Dietary practices: What does the family eat? Who prepares the food? How is food prepared?

   Family relationships: Describe the roles of your family members. Who is responsible for child rearing?

CHAPTER 3

Content Review Questions

Multiple Choice

1. c
2. b
3. d
4. d
5. a
6. a
7. a
8. a
9. d
10. c
11. a

Copyright © 2003, Mosby, Inc. All rights reserved.

12. c
13. b
14. a
15. c
16. b
17. d
18. c
19. a
20. c
21. d
22. d
23. a
24. a
25. c
26. a
27. d
28. d
29. b
30. b

Terminology Review

Matching

31. n
32. g
33. m
34. h
35. q
36. a
37. p
38. c
39. e
40. j
41. f
42. k
43. o
44. b
45. i
46. r
47. d
48. l

Copyright © 2003, Mosby, Inc. All rights reserved.

Crossword Puzzle

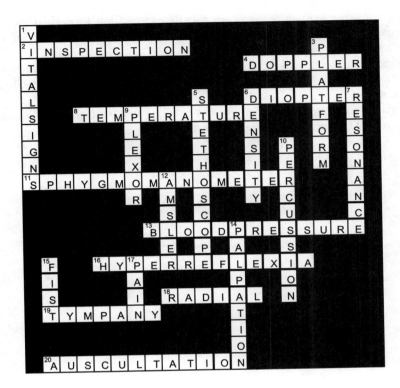

Concepts Application

Activity 1

1. Prior to the beginning of an examination
2. After touching any body fluid with or without gloves
3. After the examination

Activity 2

Area Percussed	Percussion Tone Expected
a. Stomach	tympanic
b. Sternum	flat
c. Lung of patient with emphysema	hyperresonant
d. Liver	dull
e. Lung of patient with pneumonia	dull
f. Lung of normal patient	resonant
g. Abdomen with large tumor	dull

Copyright © 2003, Mosby, Inc. All rights reserved.

Critical Thinking

1. Place Mrs. Johnson in a separate room. Wear gloves with the examination. Properly dispose of any disposable items that come into contact with the patient. Disinfect the room and any nondisposable articles after patient leaves.
2. a. Use plain soap for routine hand washing.
   b. Use an antimicrobial soap in an outbreak situation or when a specific infection is known.
3. a. Ask Mr. Helms to describe in what way his feet do not "feel right." Ask for more specific symptoms such as pain, numbness, loss of movement.
   b. The examiner should assess for the loss of protective sensation in the feet. A monofilament will help identify a patient with decreased sensation and increased risk for injury.

CHAPTER 4

Content Review Questions

Multiple Choice

1. d
2. a
3. c
4. b
5. a
6. c
7. b
8. b
9. c
10. a
11. d
12. b
13. c

Terminology Review

Matching

14. b
15. e
16. a
17. d
18. d
19. a
20. b
21. b
22. c
23. a

Copyright © 2003, Mosby, Inc. All rights reserved.

Crossword Puzzle

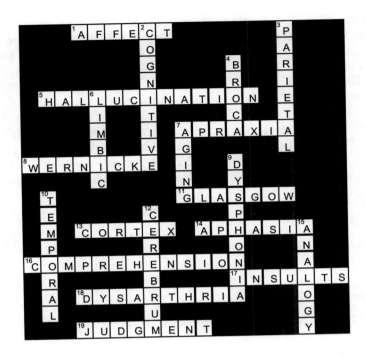

Concepts Application

1. Attention: Recite a list of numbers slowly and have the patient repeat them in the correct order. The patient should be able to correctly repeat the series of numbers.
2. Memory: Give the patient a list of items to remember and have the list repeated back after a 5-minute interval. The patient should be able to recall the items correctly.
3. Judgment: Ask the patient hypothetical questions involving situations where decisions must be made, such as finding money on the sidewalk, seeing a car on fire, etc. The patient should be able to evaluate a situation and describe an appropriate action to take in the circumstances.
4. Insight: Ask the patient to describe personal health status and reasons for consulting a health care professional. The patient should be able to demonstrate awareness and understanding of self.
5. Abstract reasoning: Recite a common proverb to the patient and request an explanation of its meaning. The patient should be able to give appropriate interpretations within his cultural frame of reference.
6. Thought processes and content: Observe the patient's pattern of thought during the interview and examination process. The patient should be logical, coherent, and goal oriented.

Case Study

1. Data deviating from normal: Patient recently lost spouse. Son says his mother has "gone downhill." Son indicates patient is no longer keeping her house clean or cooking appropriate meals. Son reports significant change in patient's personal hygiene habits. Son reports that patient becomes angry when he talks about other living options. Patient states, "You think I am helpless and want to lock me away." Patient is 78-year-old female who sits quietly during conversation. Overall hygiene clean with matted hair and clothes that do not match and are wrinkled. Overall affect is very dull; makes no eye contact with her son or the examiner.
2. The examiner should ask questions related to cognitive abilities and emotional stability.
3. The examiner should conduct a physical examination that will provide clues to her cognitive abilities as well as her emotional stability.
4. The patient may be suffering from depression.

Copyright © 2003, Mosby, Inc. All rights reserved.

Critical Thinking

1. Two types of dementia discussed in the textbook are Alzheimer's dementia and vascular dementia. Alzheimer's dementia accounts for up to 50% of dementia cases and is characterized by a severe and progressive deterioration in mental function; the rate of progression varies from individual to individual. This leads to disintegration of the personality, and eventually to complete disorientation. Vascular dementia, on the other hand, is characterized by a rapid deterioration in cognitive ability, most typically related to cerebral vascular accidents (CVAs). This deterioration in cognitive ability impairs memory, resulting in an inability to learn new information or to recall previously learned information.

2. *Personality:* Although personality does not typically change, existing personality traits may become exaggerated.
   Intellectual function: Typically, intellectual function does not deteriorate before 70 years of age, unless a disease process or medications affect it. Some individuals have problems understanding new concepts by 80 years of age.
   Problem-solving skills: There is a deterioration of problem-solving skills with aging, but it is thought that this may be a result of disuse.
   Memory: Short-term, or recent, memory typically deteriorates before distant memory.

CHAPTER 5

Content Review Questions

Multiple Choice

1. d
2. b
3. d
4. b
5. a
6. d
7. b
8. a
9. b
10. c
11. c
12. a
13. d
14. a
15. c

Terminology Review

16. head circumference
17. SMR (Sexual Maturity Rating)
18. BMI (Body Mass Index)
19. adult stature
20. Ballard Gestational Age Assessment
21. recumbent length
22. gestational age
23. infant stature

Copyright © 2003, Mosby, Inc. All rights reserved.

Matching

24. d
25. e
26. a
27. f
28. b
29. c

Crossword Puzzle

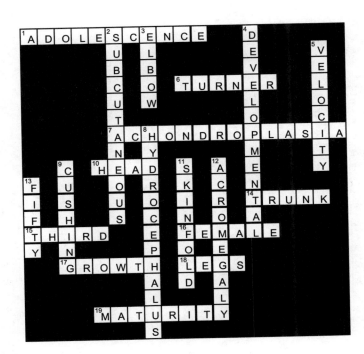

Concepts Application

1. Maturity rating score: 45
   Gestational age: 36
2. Baby Michael's length percentile: 20th
   Baby Michael's weight percentile: 30th
   Baby Michael's head circumference percentile: 50th
3. At 36 weeks gestation, Baby Michael is just slightly premature. Compared with other neonates born at 36 weeks, Michael is within a normal range of growth measurement.

Copyright © 2003, Mosby, Inc. All rights reserved.

External sign	Score				
	0	1	2	3	4
Edema	Obvious edema of hands and feet; pitting over tibia	No obvious edema of hands and feet; pitting over tibia	No edema		
Skin texture	Very thin, gelatinous	Thin and smooth	Smooth; medium thickness. Rash or superficial peeling	Slight thickening. Superficial cracking and peeling, especially of hands and feet	Thick and parchmentlike; superficial or deep cracking
Skin color	Dark red	Uniformly pink	Pale pink; variable over body	Pale; only pink over ears, lips, palms, or soles	
Skin opacity (trunk)	Numerous veins and venules clearly seen, especially over abdomen	Veins and tributaries seen	A few large vessels clearly seen over abdomen	A few large vessels seen indistinctly over abdomen	No blood vessels seen
Lanugo (over back)	No lanugo	Abundant; long and thick over whole back	Hair thinning especially over lower back	Small amount of lanugo and bald areas	At least 1/2 of back devoid of lanugo
Plantar creases	No skin creases	Faint red marks over anterior half of sole	Definite red marks over > anterior 1/2; indentations over < anterior 1/3	Indentations over > anterior 1/3	Definite deep indentations over > anterior 1/3
Nipple formation	Nipple barely visible; no areola	Nipple well defined; areola smooth and flat, diameter < 0.75 cm	Areola stippled, edge not raised, diameter < 0.75 cm	Areola stippled, edge raised, diameter > 0.75 cm	
Breast size	No breast tissue palpable	Breast tissue on one or both sides, < 0.5 cm diameter	Breast tissue both sides; one or both 0.5-1 cm	Breast tissue both sides; one or both > 1 cm	
Ear form	Pinna flat and shapeless, little or no incurving of edge	Incurving of part of edge of pinna	Partial incurving whole of upper pinna	Well-defined incurving whole of upper pinna	
Ear firmness	Pinna soft, easily folded, no recoil	Pinna soft, easily folded, slow recoil	Cartilage to edge of pinna, but soft in places, ready recoil	Pinna firm, cartilage to edge; instant recoil	
Genitals Male	Neither testis in scrotum	At least one testis high in scrotum	At least one testis right down		
Female (with hips 1/2 abducted)	Labia majora widely separated, labia minora protruding	Labia majora almost cover labia minora	Labia majora completely cover labia minora		

Copyright © 2003, Mosby, Inc. All rights reserved.

Neurologic signs	Score					
	0	1	2	3	4	5
Posture			(circled)			
Square window	90°	60°	(circled) 45°	30°	0°	
Ankle dorsiflexion	90°	75°	(circled) 45°	20°	0°	
Arm recoil	180°	(circled) 90°-180°	<90°			
Leg recoil	180°	(circled) 90°-180°	<90°			
Popliteal angle	180°	160°	(circled) 130°	110°	90°	<90°
Heel to ear				(circled)		
Scarf sign			(circled)			
Head lag		(circled)				
Ventral suspension			(circled)			

Total score	Weeks of gestation
0-9	26
10-12	27
13-16	28
17-20	29
21-24	30
25-27	31
28-31	32
32-35	33
36-39	34
40-43	35
44-46 (circled)	36 (circled)
47-50	37
51-54	38
55-58	39
59-62	40
63-65	41
66-69	42

Copyright © 2003, Mosby, Inc. All rights reserved.

CLASSIFICATION OF NEWBORNS —
BASED ON MATURITY AND INTRAUTERINE GROWTH
Symbols: X - 1st Exam   O - 2nd Exam

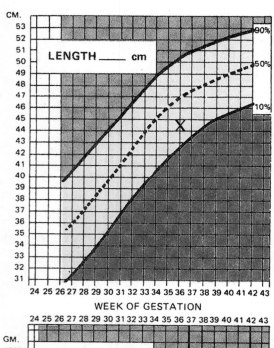

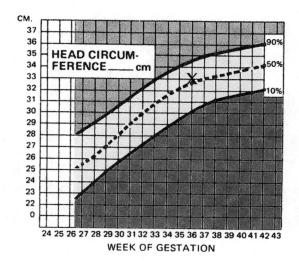

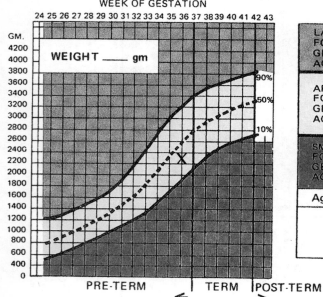

	1st Exam (X)	2nd Exam (O)
LARGE FOR GESTATIONAL AGE (LGA)		
APPROPRIATE FOR GESTATIONAL AGE (AGA)		
SMALL FOR GESTATIONAL AGE (SGA)		
Age at Exam	hrs	hrs
Signature of Examiner	_____ M.D.	_____ M.D.

Copyright © 2003, Mosby, Inc. All rights reserved.

CHAPTER 6

Content Review Questions

Multiple Choice

1. c
2. d
3. a
4. b
5. a
6. b
7. b
8. d
9. c
10. b
11. a
12. c
13. d
14. a
15. b
16. c
17. b
18. d

Terminology Review

19. body mass index
20. resting energy expenditure
21. midarm muscle circumference
22. anorexia
23. bulexaremia
24. endogenous obesity
25. Bitot's spots
26. cheilosis
27. anthropometrics
28. exogenous obesity

Copyright © 2003, Mosby, Inc. All rights reserved.

Crossword Puzzle

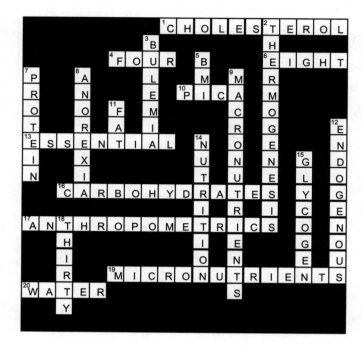

Concepts Application

Activity 1

(The formula necessary to complete this activity is from Table 6-9 in the textbook.)

15-year-old male weighing 110 pounds:	$(17.5 \times 110) + 651$	$= 2576$ kcal/day
25-year-old female weighing 142 pounds:	$(14.7 \times 142) + 496$	$= 2583$ kcal/day
32-year-old female weighing 200 pounds:	$(8.7 \times 200) + 829$	$= 2569$ kcal/day
62-year old male weighing 168 pounds:	$(13.5 \times 168) + 487$	$= 2755$ kcal/day

Activity 2

1. Desirable body weight: $5' 9" = 106 + (6 \times 9) = 160$ lbs
2. % desirable body weight: $142/160 \times 100$ $= 88.75\%$
3. % usual body weight: $142/172 \times 100$ $= 82356\%$
4. % weight change: $172 - 142/172 \times 100$ $= 17.44\%$
5. Current BMI $= 21.08$
   Previous BMI $= 25.55$
6. 10th percentile
7. Based on all the calculations, Jack has had a very significant loss in weight. A change of 17% body weight in 9-month period of time is of great concern.

CHAPTER 7

Content Review Questions

Multiple Choice

1. a
2. c

Copyright © 2003, Mosby, Inc. All rights reserved.

3. a
4. b
5. d
6. c
7. c
8. d
9. b
10. a
11. a
12. a
13. a
14. b
15. c
16. a
17. d
18. b
19. b
20. d

Terminology Review

21. confluent
22. acrocyanosis
23. reticulate
24. alopecia
25. harlequin
26. stellate
27. erythema toxicum
28. generalized
29. serpiginous
30. annular
31. Mongolian spots
32. keloid
33. morbilliform
34. ecchymosis
35. dermatomal
36. vesicle
37. petechiae
38. cutis marmorata
39. plaque

Matching

40. c
41. h
42. e
43. g
44. d
45. i
46. a
47. f
48. b

Copyright © 2003, Mosby, Inc. All rights reserved.

Crossword Puzzle

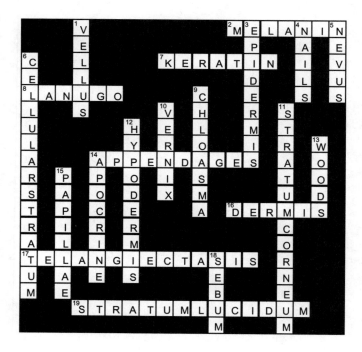

Anatomy Review

a. cuticle
b. nail plate
c. perionychium
d. lunula
e. eponychium

Concepts Application

Name of Lesion	*Example*
A. Excoriation	Abrasion, scratch, scabies
B. Fissure	Athlete's foot, cracks at corner of mouth
C. Erosion	Varicella or variola after rupture
D. Ulcer	Decubitus ulcers, stasis ulcers

Case Study

1. All data described is considered normal for the age of the patient, with the exception of the ulcerations on the lower extremities. This could be due to a number of factors, but it is definitely not within normal limits for any age.
2. Ask when he first noticed the lesions, how often he has had the lesions, and what seems to help them get better. Ask if he has any pain in his legs associated with activity.
3. Assess circulation to the feet. An ulcerated open wound that does not heal most likely indicates insufficient perfusion of blood leading to tissue anoxia. It is possible that a Doppler may be needed to assess pulses, or vascular studies may need to be considered.
4. The most common reason for this problem is insufficient perfusion. This may be the result of underlying vascular disease or heart disease; it may also be associated with diabetes.

Copyright © 2003, Mosby, Inc. All rights reserved.

Critical Thinking

1. Explain the following ABCD early signs of melanoma to Mr. Mason:

    A = Asymmetry: Melanoma lesions are asymmetrical in shape and appearance.

    B = Border: Melanoma lesions have irregular, indistinct, and sometimes notched borders.

    C = Color: Melanoma lesions tend to have uneven and variegated color. Lesions may vary from brown to pink to purple or have a mixed pigmentation.

    D = Diameter: Melanoma lesions are usually over 6 cm (2 inches) in diameter.

2. The examiner should note the following: location (where the lesion is found); distribution (isolated lesions or confluent); color; size; pattern (clustered, linear, etc.); shape; elevation (flat, raised); characteristics (hard, soft, crusty, fluid-filled, solid, draining).

CHAPTER 8

Content Review Questions

Multiple Choice

1. a
2. d
3. b
4. c
5. b
6. b
7. c
8. c
9. a
10. d
11. c
12. d
13. b
14. c
15. a

Terminology Review

Matching

16. d
17. a
18. f
19. b
20. e
21. c

Copyright © 2003, Mosby, Inc. All rights reserved.

Anatomy Review

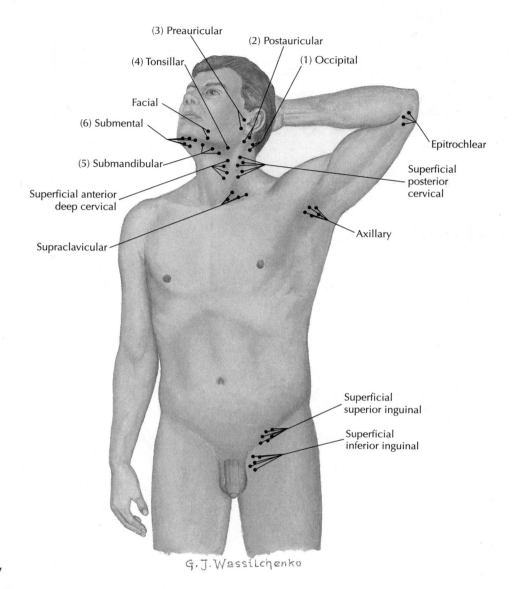

(3) Preauricular
(2) Postauricular
(4) Tonsillar
(1) Occipital
Facial
(6) Submental
Epitrochlear
(5) Submandibular
Superficial posterior cervical
Superficial anterior deep cervical
Supraclavicular
Axillary
Superficial superior inguinal
Superficial inferior inguinal

G. J. Wassilchenko

Case Study

1. Data deviating from normal: fatigue/weakness, enlarged lymph nodes.
2. Ask whether there is tenderness to the lymph nodes. Ask whether the patient has been ill recently. Ask whether he has had recent weight loss, whether he has been eating properly, and whether he has been getting adequate sleep.
3. Assess lymph nodes in neck, axilla, arm, and groin. Compare palpable lymph nodes for symmetry. Note the size, consistency, mobility, borders, and tenderness of lymph nodes.
4. Enlarged lymph nodes could be the result of a recent viral infection or a more serious problem such as a lymphoma or malignancy.

Critical Thinking

1. The nine S's are size, shape, surface characteristics, site, symptoms, softness, squeezability, spread, and sensations.
2. Compared with the adult, the lymph system of the infant or small child is proportionally much larger (the thymus, in particular, is quite large). Lymph nodes are normally readily palpable. After puberty, the lymph nodes become small and much less pronounced. The thymus shrinks to a point where it is not assessed. By the time the adult reaches late adult years, the lymph nodes become very small and have limited function. The nodes become fibrotic and fatty and become impaired in ability to resist infection.

Copyright © 2003, Mosby, Inc. All rights reserved.

CHAPTER 9

Content Review Questions

Multiple Choice

1. c
2. a
3. b
4. d
5. d
6. a
7. b
8. d
9. c
10. a
11. d
12. b
13. d
14. a
15. c

Terminology Review

Matching

16. d
17. c
18. a
19. e
20. b

Crossword Puzzle

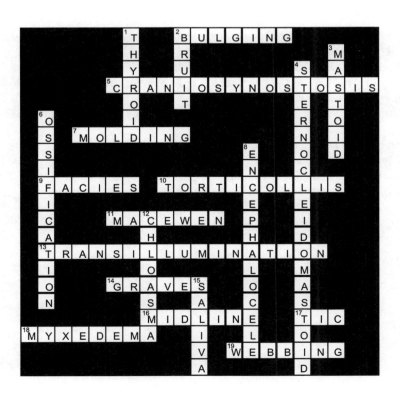

Copyright © 2003, Mosby, Inc. All rights reserved.

Anatomy Review

a. trachea
b. jugular vein
c. cricoid cartilage
d. hyoid bone
e. carotid artery
f. thyroid gland
g. lymph node

Concepts Application

System or Structure	Hyperthyroidism	Hypothyroidism
Weight	Weight loss	Weight gain
Emotional state	Nervous; irritable	Lethargic; disinterested
Temperature preference	Prefers cool climate	Prefers warm climate
Hair	Fine hair with hair loss	Coarse hair that breaks easily
Skin	Warm skin with hyperpigmentation	Coarse, dry, scaling skin at pressure points
Neck	Goiter	No goiter
Gastrointestinal	Increased peristalsis; increased frequency of bowel movements	Decreased peristalsis; constipation
Eyes	Puffiness in periorbital region	Proptosis; lid retraction

Case Study

1. Data deviating from normal: Patient complains of severe recurring headache. Nasal stuffiness occurs with headache. Nothing seems to help headache.
2. Get more information about the headache, including the following:
   Pattern of headaches: How often do the headaches occur? At what time of day do they occur? How would you characterize the onset of the headaches (gradual vs. sudden)?
   Characteristics of headache: Where is the pain? What is the pain like? How long does the pain last? How severe is the pain?
   Precipitating factors: What brings the headache on?
   Treatment: What has Rob done to try to treat these headaches?
   History: Is there any past or recent history of trauma to the head?
3. Assess range of motion in the neck, if possible, and attempt to palpate the neck for lymph nodes.

Copyright © 2003, Mosby, Inc. All rights reserved.

Critical Thinking

1. Percussion of the head and neck is not routinely performed. Percussion over the sinuses is applicable if the examiner suspects sinusitis in order to determine whether tenderness exists. There is also some evidence that individuals with hyperparathyroidism will have a low-pitched sound to percussion of the skull (as opposed to a high-pitched sound normally expected).

2. Like percussion, auscultation of the head is not routinely performed. However, if a vascular anomaly of the brain is suspected, bruits might be heard. It is best to listen over the eyes, the temporal region, and just below the occiput of the skull.

CHAPTER 10

Content Review Questions

Multiple Choice

1. d
2. b
3. a
4. c
5. b
6. a
7. a
8. c
9. d
10. d
11. b
12. a
13. c
14. b
15. c
16. a
17. a
18. d
19. b
20. b

Terminology Review

Matching

21. c
22. b
23. e
24. a
25. d
26. g
27. f

Copyright © 2003, Mosby, Inc. All rights reserved.

Crossword Puzzle

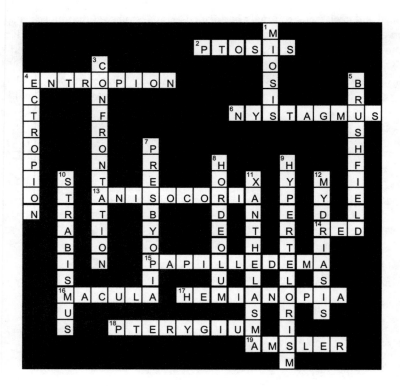

Concepts Application

Activity 1

Location: Lesion is 1 1/2 DD at clock position of 2:30.
Length: 3/4 DD
Width: 1/2 DD

Activity 2

Structure	What Should Be Examined
1. Eyelid	Observe position of eyelids when eyes are open and when eyelids are closed completely. Inspect for eversion or inversion of lids, presence of nodules.
2. Conjunctiva	Inspect for inflammation, presence of foreign body, increased erythema or exudate. Observe for pterygium.
3. Cornea	Assess corneal sensitivity. Note lipid deposits on cornea. Assess clarity.
4. Iris and pupil	Check for response to light and accommodation. Estimate pupillary sizes; compare them for equality.
5. Lens	Inspect for clarity—lens should appear transparent.
6. Sclera	Check for color of sclera and for pigmentation.
7. Lacrimal apparatus	Inspect and palpate. Check for tearing.

Case Study

1. Data deviating from normal: history of poorly controlled diabetes; sudden change in vision; significant visual acuity findings; ophthalmoscope findings; new vessels and presence of hemorrhage vessels.
2. Ask the patient whether he has pain. Ask whether the change in vision has been gradual and progressive or intermittent. Ask whether he has any other symptoms associated with the change in vision, such as intolerance to light. Ask him whether he currently wears contact lenses or glasses. Ask how long he has had diabetes.

Copyright © 2003, Mosby, Inc. All rights reserved.

3. It is important to determine the last visual acuity results to compare with the current one.
4. Andy has one major problem at this point that affects multiple areas. If he loses his vision, the impact on functional abilities will be tremendous and will include (but not be limited to) safety, self-care activities, management of his diabetes, independence, and employment.

Critical Thinking

1. General inspection of external structures of the eye should be done. Visual acuity should be checked with a Snellen E chart. A red-reflex should be checked; corneal light and reflex/cover-uncover should also be done. Finally, examination of extraocular movements and cranial nerves III, IV, and VI should be done, including asking the child to follow through the six cardinal fields of gaze.
2. The first clue is the size; retinal arteries are about 1/4 narrower than retinal veins. The second difference is the color. Arteries appear as a very light red color and may have a narrow band of light reflex in the center. Veins, on the other hand, are darker in color and do not have a band of light reflex.

CHAPTER 11

Content Review Questions

Multiple Choice

1. a
2. c
3. c
4. a
5. d
6. b
7. c
8. b
9. d
10. a
11. c
12. a
13. b
14. d
15. b

Terminology Review

16. Nylen Barany
17. Koplik's spots
18. Darwin tubercle
19. malocclusion
20. Epstein's pearls

Matching

21. c
22. d
23. b
24. e
25. a

Copyright © 2003, Mosby, Inc. All rights reserved.

Crossword Puzzle

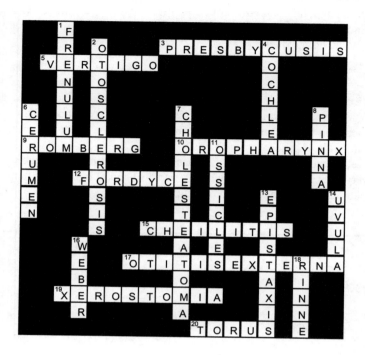

Anatomy Review

a. malleus
b. incus
c. stapes
d. tympanic membrane
e. cochlea
f. cochlear duct

Case Study

1. Data deviating from normal: fever; complaints of ear pain; presence of drainage in ear canal; TM perforation; reduction of hearing in left ear; quiet affect; limited talking.
2. Ask what treatment the child has received for the ear pain from the medicine man in the past. Ask the mother whether she has ever seen drainage from the ear with past problems. Ask whether the child has been treated at a hospital or clinic for ear pain in the past.
3. If possible, complete a Rinne test. A full hearing assessment with an audiometer is probably in order as well. Also, complete a developmental assessment.
4. Primary problems: The child has obvious hearing impairment. There is also some evidence that there may be a developmental delay—possibly associated with the hearing loss.

Critical Thinking

1. To differentiate redness associated with crying versus otitis media, look for other clinical signs: primarily bulging and mobility of the tympanic membrane.
2. Obstructive sleep apnea is caused by a relaxation of the muscles in the nasopharynx, hypopharynx, and pharynx during sleep. This causes an obstruction in the airflow leading to progressive hypercapnia, hypoxemia, and increased pulmonary arterial pressures.

Copyright © 2003, Mosby, Inc. All rights reserved.

CHAPTER 12

Content Review Questions

Multiple Choice

1. d
2. c
3. b
4. d
5. a
6. c
7. a
8. a
9. c
10. d
11. c
12. a
13. b
14. a
15. c
16. b
17. d
18. b
19. d
20. a
21. d
22. b
23. b
24. c
25. a

Terminology Review

Matching

26. f
27. h
28. a
29. j
30. b
31. b
32. l
33. c
34. k
35. d
36. m
37. g
38. e

Copyright © 2003, Mosby, Inc. All rights reserved.

Crossword Puzzle

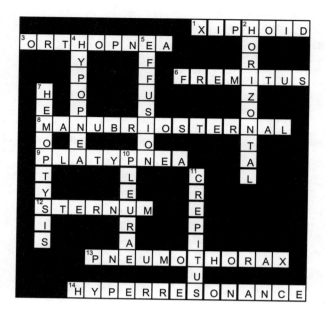

Concepts Application

Activity 1

Conditions	Examination Technique
Tuberculosis vs. pneumonia	Check sputum: Bacterial pneumonia classically is greenish yellow; TB typically is bloody.
Pneumothorax vs. atelectasis	Percussion: Atelectasis typically is dull; pneumothorax has hyperresonance.
Pneumonia vs. pleural effusion	Check fremitus: Pleural effusion is associated with decreased fremitus; pneumonia is associated with increased fremitus.
Asthma vs. emphysema	Auscultate breath sounds: Asthma classically has wheezes; emphysema is likely to have fine to moderate crackles.

Activity 2

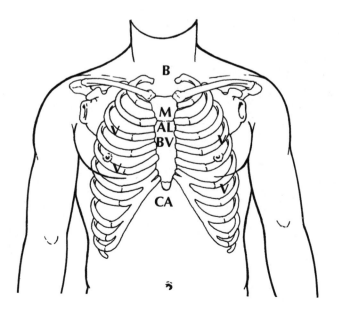

Copyright © 2003, Mosby, Inc. All rights reserved.

Case Study

1. Data deviating from normal: history of shortness of breath; limitation in activity; interrupted sleep (requiring pillows); smoking history; labored breathing with tachypnea; presence of cyanosis; underweight/protruding ribs; increased AP diameter; reduced chest wall movement; diminished tactile fremitus; adventitious breath sounds; and diminished breath sounds.
2. Ask about chest pain with shortness of breath. Ask about the presence of cough. Ask how old patient was when she started smoking and how long she has been smoking as much as she currently is.
3. Assess oxygen saturation, body weight, and rhythm of breathing pattern. Assess for presence of retractions. Percuss the chest for tone and diaphragmatic excursion.
4. Primary problems for this patient include respiratory/oxygenation problems and nutrition problems. Patients who are short of breath have difficulty maintaining adequate nutrition.

Critical Thinking

1. He has a 9-year history at 1/3 pack a day (3 pack years); a 15-year history at 1/2 pack a day (7 1/2 pack years); and 32-year history of 1 pack a day (32 pack years) for a total of 42 1/2 pack-year history.
2. These symptoms are consistent with tuberculosis. High-risk groups include Native Americans and immigrants from Mexico. He should be placed in airborne isolation until diagnosis is made.
3. Ask what has changed. The mother said the family moved recently; ask about the new home and environment, possible irritants within the new home. Also ask about ventilation and air conditioning, exposure to smoke and pets in or around the home.

CHAPTER 13

Content Review Questions

Multiple Choice

1. c
2. b
3. a
4. a
5. c
6. a
7. b
8. c
9. c
10. b
11. b
12. c
13. c
14. a
15. a
16. c
17. a
18. b
19. d
20. c
21. a
22. d
23. d
24. b
25. c

Copyright © 2003, Mosby, Inc. All rights reserved.

Terminology Review

Crossword Puzzle

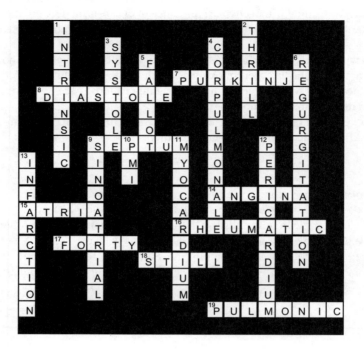

Anatomy Review

a. inferior vena cava
b. tricuspid valve
c. pulmonic valve
d. right pulmonary artery
e. right subclavian artery
f. superior vena cava
g. right common carotid artery
h. left common carotid artery
i. left subclavian artery
j. left pulmonary artery
k. aortic valve
l. mitral valve
m. aorta

Concepts Application

Valve	*Where Would You Auscultate?*
Tricuspid valve	4th left intercostal space
Mitral valve	5th left intercostal space
Aortic valve	2nd right intercostal space
Pulmonic valve	2nd left intercostal space

Case Study

1. Data deviating from normal: complaint of shortness of breath; complaint of fatigue that interferes with routine activities; complaint of sleeping difficulty; labored breathing with elevated respiratory rate, pulse rate, and blood pressure; pitting edema in lower extremities; frothy-looking phlegm.

Copyright © 2003, Mosby, Inc. All rights reserved.

2. Complete a symptom analysis on the shortness of breath and fatigue. Ask the patient whether he has symptoms associated with chest pain, cough, or nocturia. Ask the patient about cardiovascular history.

3. Perform a precordial assessment including inspection, percussion, palpation, and auscultation.

4. First, this patient has a perfusion problem. The decrease in cardiac output reduces the perfusion of oxygenated blood to the body, causing the symptoms of fatigue. Second, this patient has an oxygenation problem. Since the heart is not pumping efficiently, blood is backing up in the pulmonary bed, resulting in pulmonary edema. Pulmonary edema interferes with the exchange of oxygen and carbon dioxide in the lungs.

Critical Thinking

1. This finding, without other symptoms, may not be relevant. However, children who have congenital heart defects tend to squat frequently because squatting relieves dyspnea.

2. Look for polyarthritis, chorea, erythema marginatum, subcutaneous nodules, arthralgia, an increase in the sedimentation rate, or leukocytosis.

3. Diabetes will cause an increase in basement membrane of capillaries, which make these vessels narrower. Narrowing contributes to hypertension and impaired perfusion of the lower extremities.

CHAPTER 14

Content Review Questions

Multiple Choice

1. c
2. b
3. a
4. a
5. c
6. a
7. b
8. c
9. c
10. b
11. b
12. c
13. c
14. a
15. a
16. c
17. a
18. b
19. d
20. c
21. a
22. d
23. d
24. b
25. c

Copyright © 2003, Mosby, Inc. All rights reserved.

Terminology Review

Crossword Puzzle

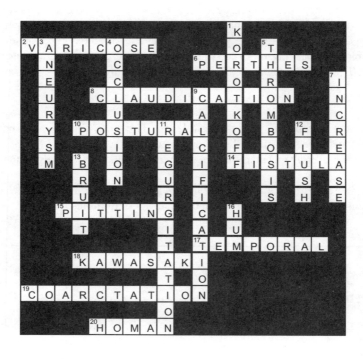

Case Study

1. Data deviating from normal: changes in color and temperature of the hands; exertional dyspnea; presence of dark lesion on the fifth right finger.
2. Complete a symptom analysis on the circulation in the hands and the dyspnea. Ask the patient whether the pain and color changes vary with activity or environmental changes; also ask how long the episodes of pain last and how frequently they occur. Ask the patient about other symptoms of dyspnea that may be interfering with activities of daily living.
3. Perform further neurologic assessment of the hands, obtain chest film and pulmonary function studies; complete evaluation for connective tissue disease including appropriate labwork (ESR, ANA titer, and chemistry studies).
4. This patient has a circulatory problem that is most likely secondary to connective tissue disease and exacerbated by smoking. The intermittent spasms of the arterioles in the fingers causes pallor and the accompanying decrease in circulation produces claudication. The appearance of impending ulceration on the finger signals the need for monitoring of the patient's circulatory status. The patient may develop spasms in the nose and tongue, and she should be educated about this possibility and encouraged to report any changes in her circulatory status.

Critical Thinking

1. The symptoms suggest venous thrombosis and the patient is at risk for pulmonary embolus.
2. Blood pressure can change with position changes by the mother. Hypotension is frequently noted during the third trimester when the patient in supine. This is secondary to venous occlusion of the vena cava and resulting impaired venous return. In addition blood tends to stagnate in the lower extremities as a result of occlusion of the pelvic veins and the inferior vena cava created by the growing uterus.

Copyright © 2003, Mosby, Inc. All rights reserved.

CHAPTER 15

Content Review Questions

Multiple Choice

1. a
2. c
3. a
4. b
5. a
6. c
7. c
8. b
9. d
10. b
11. d
12. c
13. b
14. a
15. b

Terminology Review

Matching

16. d
17. e
18. b
19. a
20. c

Crossword Puzzle

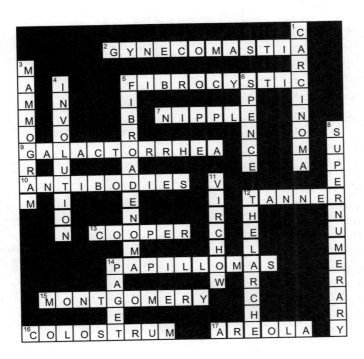

Copyright © 2003, Mosby, Inc. All rights reserved.

Concepts Application

(a)

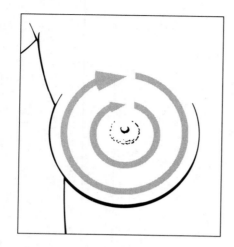

(b)

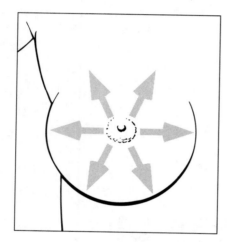

(c)

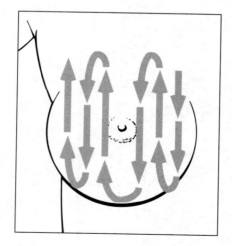

Copyright © 2003, Mosby, Inc. All rights reserved.

Case Study

1. Data deviating from normal: Patient has a history of nontender breast lump, noticeable for about 9 months. Mass has increased in size over 9 months. Risk factors include early onset of menarche and the fact that the patient is childless. Palpable lump is present in the left upper outer quadrant. Dimpling noted on left breast. Left nipple is retracted. Bloody discharge is noted from nipple when squeezed.
2. Ask about personal or family history of breast disease. Ask patient whether she does regular breast self-exams. Ask whether she has ever had a mammogram. Ask about location of lump. Ask whether lump is tender now. Ask whether she has noticed nipple discharge. Ask about changes in the lump size in relation to menstrual cycle.
3. Inspect the areolae. Besides location, the following characteristics must be assessed with a breast mass: size, shape, consistency, tenderness, mobility, and borders. Palpate the axilla. It is especially important to note any lumps or masses in the left axilla.
4. Primary problems: This patient has a very suspicious breast mass consistent with malignancy. She also seems to be in denial with this problem.

Critical Thinking

1. Risk factors for breast cancer: Patient is female. She is over the age of 40. She had an early onset of menarche. She had her first and only child at the age of 36. She has a strong family history of breast cancer. Although it cannot be predicted who will and will not develop breast cancer, this woman certainly has very strong risk factors.
2. Offer the following instructions: Perform breast self-examination every month—at the same time every month. Undress and stand in front of a mirror. Look at your breasts in the following three positions: (1) standing with hands on hips; (2) standing with arms extended above your head; and (3) leaning forward with your hands outstretched. Watch for any changes in the way your breast appears, such as a dimpling, puckering, changes in size. Palpate your breasts. Raise your left arm over your head. Starting at the nipple of the left breast, firmly press the fingers from your right hand in a circular motion, working outward and feeling every part of your breast. You are feeling for any lump or mass. After you palpate your breast, squeeze the nipple and look for any discharge. Repeat this procedure with other breast. You may do this procedure standing and/or lying down. If you feel any lumps or see any discharge from your nipple, you should contact your primary health provider.

CHAPTER 16

Content Review Questions

Multiple Choice

1. d
2. c
3. b
4. c
5. a
6. d
7. b
8. c
9. d
10. c
11. a
12. c
13. d
14. d
15. d
16. d
17. b
18. a

Copyright © 2003, Mosby, Inc. All rights reserved.

19. b
20. a
21. c
22. c
23. a
24. b
25. c

Terminology Review

Matching

26. d
27. c
28. a
29. e
30. f
31. b

Crossword Puzzle

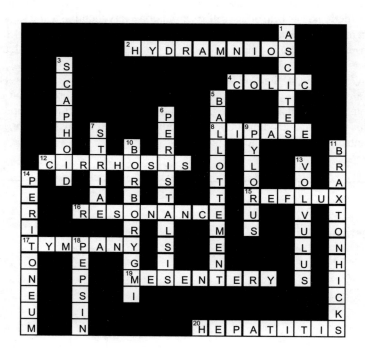

Copyright © 2003, Mosby, Inc. All rights reserved.

Anatomy Review

Activity 1

a. liver
b. gallbladder
c. colon
d. appendix
e. small intestine
f. pancreas
g. stomach
h. spleen

Activity 2

Structure	Quadrant	Region
Appendix	right lower quadrant	right inguinal
Colon	ascending/transverse RUQ transverse and descending LUQ ascending RLQ descending LLQ	ascending—right lumbar transverse—umbilical descending—left lumbar
Gallbladder	right upper quadrant	right hypochondriac
Liver	right upper quadrant	right hypochondriac (right lobe) epigastric
Pancreas	left upper quadrant (body) right upper quadrant (head)	epigastric left hypochondriac (tail)
Small intestine	right lower quadrant left lower quadrant	umbilical hypogastric
Spleen	left upper quadrant	left hypochondriac
Stomach	left upper quadrant	epigastric umbilical

Copyright © 2003, Mosby, Inc. All rights reserved.

Concepts Application

Condition	Type of Pain	Abdominal Signs	Associated Symptoms or Findings
Peritonitis	Sudden or gradual onset of generalized or localized pain described as dull or severe; increased pain with deep inspiration	+ Markle's sign + Rosving's sign + Blumberg's sign	Shallow respirations; nausea and vomiting; guarding; decreased bowel sounds; + obturator and iliopsoas tests
Cholecystitis	RUQ and epigastric pain that refers to right subscapular region	+ Murphy's sign	Anorexia, nausea, vomiting, fever, abdominal rigidity
Ectopic pregnancy	Lower quadrant pain that may refer to the shoulder—agonizing pain with rupture	+ Cullen's sign + Kehr's sign	Tender cervix, discharge, dyspareunia, symptoms of pregnancy; spotting, hypogastric tenderness, mass on bimanual pelvic exam; with rupture: shock, rigid abdominal wall, distention
Pancreatitis	Sudden and dramatic LUQ, umbilical, or epigastric pain that may be referred to L shoulder	+ Grey-Turner's sign + Cullen's sign	Fever, epigastric tenderness, vomiting
Renal calculi	Intense flank pain extending to groin and genitals	+ Kehr's sign	Fever, hematuria

Case Study

1. Data deviating from normal: abdominal pain (progressively worse); loss of appetite and nausea; guarded position; hot skin, possibly indicating fever; absence of bowel sounds; pain to palpation and guarding RLQ; positive rebound tenderness in RLQ.
2. Ask patient about vomiting with her nausea. Ask about her menstrual cycle (LMP), about the possibility of pregnancy, and about bowel elimination (last BM) and the appearance of her stool.
3. Check vital signs (of particular interest is temperature). Auscultate for arterial bruits and venous hums. Percuss kidney for CVA tenderness. Perform iliopsoas muscle test and obturator muscle test.
4. Primary problems: Patient demonstrates symptoms consistent with acute abdominal condition, very likely appendicitis. A complete blood count would be helpful.

Critical Thinking

1. Listen to the abdomen for bruits in the aortic, renal, iliac, and femoral arteries. A bruit in these arteries may indicate stenosis or an aneurysm. Listen in the umbilical area for a venous hum (soft, low-pitched, and continuous). A venous hum suggests increased collateral circulation between portal and systemic venous systems and may indicate portal hypertension. A friction rub is high-pitched and may be heard in association with respiration. This may indicate inflammation of peritoneal surface from tumor or infection.
2. You will ask Mr. Cane to place his hand on top of his abdomen. You will then place one of your hands on the side of his abdomen near the flank; use the other hand to tap on the other side of the abdomen. It is considered positive if the tap causes a fluid wave through the abdomen that is felt by your hand on the side of his abdomen.
3. Expected findings unique to pregnancy include decreased bowel sounds, linea nigra, striae, diastasis recti, quickening, and venous pattern.

Copyright © 2003, Mosby, Inc. All rights reserved.

CHAPTER 17

Content Review Questions

Multiple Choice

1. c
2. a
3. b
4. b
5. a
6. d
7. b
8. c
9. d
10. b
11. b
12. a
13. d
14. d
15. b
16. b
17. d
18. c
19. a
20. c

Terminology Review

Matching

21. O, E
22. C
23. O, E
24. E
25. C
26. O, C
27. C
28. O, E
29. E
30. C
31. d
32. e
33. a
34. f
35. g
36. b

Copyright © 2003, Mosby, Inc. All rights reserved.

Concepts Application

Position	Description	Advantages/Disadvantages
Knee-chest	Patient lies on side with both knees bent, top leg closer to chest.	May be difficult or uncomfortable for patient who is obese or has very large breasts.
Diamond-shape	Patient lies on back with knees bent so that legs are spread flat and heels meet at the foot of table.	Patient must be able to lie flat on back for this position and have flexible legs.
Obstetric stirrups	Patient lies on back near foot of bed with legs supported under the knees in obstetrical stirrups.	These offer more support than traditional foot stirrups.
M-shape	Patient lies on back, knees bent apart, feet resting on the exam table close to buttocks.	Entire body can be supported by the table.
V-shape	Patient lies on back with legs straightened out and spread wide to either side of the table.	Assistance is needed to maintain this position.

Case Study

1. Data deviating from normal: History suggests some type of acute inflammation. History is also suggestive of multiple sex contacts; primary partner has multiple sex contacts. Mass with inflammation, discharge, and extreme pain to palpation needs further evaluation.
2. Ask patient about past sexual history and associated medical problems, if any. Identification of protection (or lack of) would also be helpful.
3. A culture of discharge should be obtained for evaluation. If patient is too uncomfortable for internal examination, this may need to be delayed until the inflammation has resolved.
4. Based on symptoms and findings, patient most likely has an acute abscess of the Bartholin's gland. This is frequently associated with gonococcal or staphylococcal infection.

Critical Thinking

1. The key concept when performing an examination on a patient with visual impairment is to explain everything that is to occur, as well as what you want the patient to do. Prior to the examination, the patient should be given an opportunity to explore the instruments used during the examination.

   Other general concepts to keep in mind include introducing yourself, remembering to identify others who enter the room, and letting the patient know when others are leaving the room. Also, orient the patient to the surroundings. This patient may need assistance in getting into the proper position for examination.
2. The history is vital to obtain. At this age, it will be necessary to talk with her while her parents are out of the room. Questions should be simple, gentle, and nonjudgmental. These will greatly improve the accuracy of the information she is willing to share. There is no one set rule to determine the age when a full examination of the genitalia is necessary. However, a good rule of thumb is that if they are sexually active, examinations should be done. The examination should be carried out similarly to that of an adult.

Copyright © 2003, Mosby, Inc. All rights reserved.

CHAPTER 18

Content Review Questions

Multiple Choice

1. d
2. a
3. c
4. b
5. b
6. c
7. a
8. c
9. a
10. a
11. c
12. c
13. d
14. b
15. d

Terminology Review

Crossword Puzzle

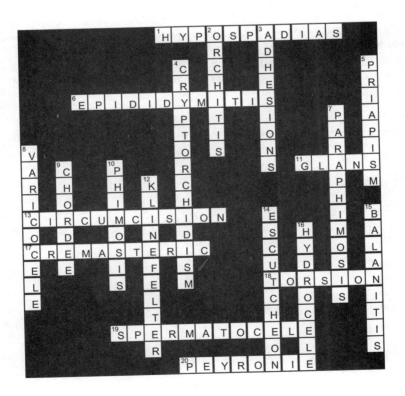

Copyright © 2003, Mosby, Inc. All rights reserved.

Matching

16. d
17. b
18. e
19. a
20. c
21. c
22. d
23. a
24. b
25. e
26. e

Case Study

1. Data deviating from normal: Protrusion or mass is noted in left groin area. History suggests possibly a hernia.
2. Discuss level of discomfort and other related symptoms. Determine whether there is history of this problem.
3. Examiner needs to determine whether this hernia is reducible. If it is nonreducible, it may require prompt surgical intervention. Also, full examination of genitalia is in order.
4. Based on symptoms and findings, the patient most likely has a direct inguinal hernia.

Critical Thinking

1. Discuss why genital self-examination is done: To screen for testicular cancer and to identify sexually transmitted diseases. Discuss how to perform genital self-examination. This should include the following: Inspection of the tip for evidence of swelling, sores, or discharge; palpation of the entire shaft of the penis from base to glans to feel for lumps or tenderness; and examination of the scrotum for color, texture, and presence of lesions. Patient should also palpate his scrotum for presence of lumps, swelling, or tenderness.
2. Be sure one of the child's parents is present. Explain to the child what you must do and why (to be sure all his body parts are healthy). It may be necessary for the parent(s) to reassure the child that it is OK for the examiner to see his "privates."

CHAPTER 19

Content Review Questions

Multiple Choice

1. a
2. b
3. c
4. d
5. a
6. a
7. b
8. d
9. a
10. d
11. b
12. c
13. d
14. d
15. c

Copyright © 2003, Mosby, Inc. All rights reserved.

16. d
17. b
18. c
19. a
20. b

Terminology Review

Matching

21. b
22. f
23. d
24. g
25. a
26. e
27. c

Concepts Application

Screening Method	*What It Reflects*	*What Results Mean*	*When It Is Indicated*
DRE	The size and character of the prostate gland	Cancer with prostate may feel hard and have irregular nodules.	Part of periodic health screening for all men over age 50 or in men over age 40 with positive risk factors.
PSA	Glycoprotein produced by prostate tissue	PSA < 4 ng/ml: normal PSA < 4-10 ng/ml: borderline PSA > 10 ng/ml: high The higher the PSA level, the more likely cancer exists. However, men with prostate CA can have borderline to low results.	PSA routine screening in conjunction with DRE in all men over age 50 or in men over age 40 with positive risk factors.
PSA velocity	Measurement of rising PSA level over time.	Rapid rise of PSA levels may suggest prostate cancer.	Used when PSA level is in borderline range.
Free PSA ratio	Measurement of the ratio of unbound (free) to bound PSA	A low unbound (free) PSA ratio suggests increased chance that prostate cancer is present.	Used when PSA level is in borderline range.
Biopsy	Sample of prostate tissue is taken for pathologic analysis	Normal tissue: no disease or benign enlargement. Abnormal or malignant tissue in presence of prostate CA.	Recommended when (1) PSA level is in high range, (2) PSA is in borderline range with abnormal DRE findings, or (3) PSA is borderline with a low free PSA ratio.
TRUS	Ultrasound of the prostate; can measure prostate volume and shape/size	Is able to indicate areas of the prostate that require biopsy.	Used when PSA level is in borderline range.

Copyright © 2003, Mosby, Inc. All rights reserved.

Case Study

1. Data deviating from normal: sensation of rectal fullness; rectal bleeding; blood in stool; palpable mass in the rectum; weight loss; enlargement of prostate.
2. Ask patient about changes in bowel elimination pattern or changes in the appearance of the stools (besides presence of blood). Ask about abdominal discomfort or distention. Ask about problems with urination (problems with starting or force of stream). Ask about sexual history.
3. Examination should include guaiac test and inguinal lymph node assessment. As part of the abdominal assessment, examiner should specifically consider the possibility of pelvic or abdominal masses.
4. Patient has an enlarged prostate and a rectal mass. They may be interrelated or completely independent of one another. Further diagnostic testing is indicated.

Critical Thinking

1. The symptoms have some similarity, but findings will be different.
   Acute prostatitis: The patient will have an inflamed prostate; therefore, the prostate will be tender and the patient will likely have a fever. Symptoms of obstruction develop more quickly than with the other two problems. With palpation, the prostate will be tender and possibly asymmetric. Additionally, the seminal vesicles may be dilated and tender to palpation.
   Benign prostate hypertrophy: Symptoms will develop gradually, with complaints of hesitancy, decreased force of stream, dribbling, and incomplete emptying of the bladder. With palpation, the prostate will feel rubbery, symmetric, and enlarged.
   Prostatic carcinoma: The symptoms of obstruction gradually occur. With palpation, the prostate is hard and irregular and feels asymmetric; the median sulcus is obliterated.
2. Some of the questions you could ask include:
   When did bleeding start?
   How much bleeding have you noticed?
   When/where do you see the bleeding?
   What does the blood look like?
   Do you have any other symptoms associated with the bleeding such as pain, gas, cramping, weight loss, etc.?
   What do you think is causing the bleeding?

CHAPTER 20

Content Review Questions

Multiple Choice

1. d
2. a
3. c
4. b
5. c
6. d
7. c
8. d
9. b
10. d
11. a
12. d
13. b
14. c
15. b
16. a

Copyright © 2003, Mosby, Inc. All rights reserved.

17. c
18. a
19. b
20. c

Terminology Review

Crossword Puzzle

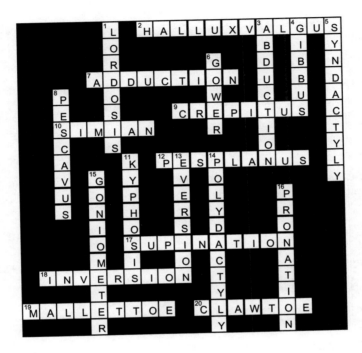

Matching

21. h
22. e
23. b
24. h
25. b
26. f
27. d
28. a
29. e
30. c
31. g

Copyright © 2003, Mosby, Inc. All rights reserved.

Concepts Application

Activity 1

Symptoms/Assessment Findings	Problem to Consider
Heberden's nodes and Bouchard's nodes noted on hands	Osteoarthritis
Low back pain that radiates to buttocks and posterior thigh, with tenderness over the spine	Lumbar disk herniation
Heat, redness, swelling, and tenderness to the metatarsophalangeal joint	Gouty arthritis of the great toe
Subcutaneous nodules on the forearm near the elbow	Rheumatoid arthritis
Tenderness, swelling, and boggy sensation with palpation along the grooves of the olecranon process; increased pain with pronation and supination	Epicondylitis or tendinitis
A child with muscle atrophy and symptoms of progressive muscle weakness	Muscular dystrophy
A child complaining of pain in the elbow and wrist; will not move his or her arm; maintains arm in a flexed and pronated position	Radial head subluxation

Activity 2

Developmental Task	Expected Age	Gross Motor or Fine Motor
Holds crayon; scribbles spontaneously.	18 months	Fine motor
Sits with shaky posture; uses tripod position; raises abdomen off table when prone.	6 months	Gross motor
When supine, puts hands together; holds hands in front of face.	3 months	Fine motor
Builds a four-block tower; dumps a raisin from a bottle.	30 months	Fine motor
Walks alone well; sits self in chair.	15 months	Gross motor
Rolls from prone to side position; slight head lag when pulled to sitting position.	3 months	Gross motor
Hops on one foot; catches bounced ball; walks heel-to-toe.	5 years	Gross motor
Reaches and picks up an object; plays with toes.	5 months	Fine motor
Points with one finger.	10 months	Fine motor
Begins creeping; stands, holding on, when placed in position.	9 months	Gross motor

Case Study

1. Data deviating from normal: diagnosis of RA; significant joint pain; limitations in self-care activities; limitations in socialization; difficulty with posture and gait; deformities to joints; tender, inflamed joints with palpation; subcutaneous nodules at the ulnar surface of the elbows.
2. Ask the patient what medications she is taking for the RA. Find out whether she is involved with any other nonpharmaceutical therapies. Ask her whether these things help or make a difference. Ask whether she has any assistive devices that she uses and/or whether she receives any assistance with self-care activities.
3. Examiner should perform documentation of ROM in various joints. Use of a goniometer would be particularly helpful.
4. Self-care activities, pain, social isolation

Copyright © 2003, Mosby, Inc. All rights reserved.

Critical Thinking

1. Muscle strain results if a muscle is stretched or torn beyond its functional capacity. A sprain is a stretching or tearing of a supporting ligament of a joint. A fracture is a partial or complete break in the continuity of the bone. Since the injury involves the joint, muscle strain is not likely. Both fractures and sprains are associated with pain and swelling and can have a bluish discoloration, so it is not always easy to differentiate these. If Mark had walked in with weight bearing on the affected ankle, it is doubtful that a fracture resulted; if he was unable to bear weight at all, it could be a fracture or a severe sprain; thus, an x-ray is usually the final diagnostic indicator.

2. A dislocation of the radial head, or radial head subluxation, is caused by jerking the arm upward while the elbow is flexed. This can occur by someone pulling on a child's arms during play or even while dressing a child. The parents must understand how this injury occurred and be taught to avoid arm-pulling activities.

CHAPTER 21

Content Review Questions

Multiple Choice

1. c
2. a
3. b
4. d
5. c
6. a
7. c
8. b
9. b
10. a
11. b
12. b
13. c
14. c
15. d
16. d
17. d
18. a
19. c
20. a

Copyright © 2003, Mosby, Inc. All rights reserved.

Terminology Review

Crossword Puzzle

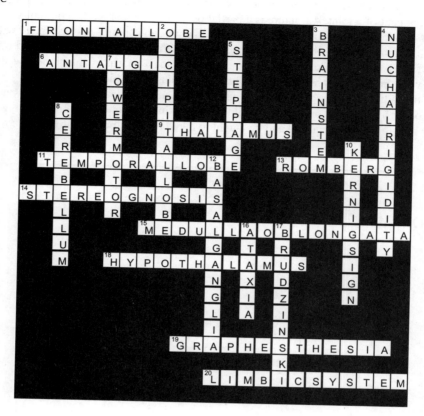

Anatomy Review

Activity 1

a. pituitary gland
b. optic chiasma
c. hypothalamus
d. corpus callosum
e. cerebrum
f. skin
g. superior sagittal sinus
h. thalamus
i. skull
j. dura mater
k. galea aponeurotica
l. tentorium cerebelli
m. midbrain
n. cerebellum
o. pons
p. medulla oblongata

Activity 2

a. cerebellum
b. cerebral peduncle
c. hypothalamus

Copyright © 2003, Mosby, Inc. All rights reserved.

d. thalamus
e. cerebrum
f. olfactory
g. optic
h. pituitary
i. oculomotor
j. trochlear
k. trigeminal
l. abducens
m. facial
n. acoustic
o. glossopharyngeal
p. vagus
q. spinal accessory
r. hypoglossal

Concepts Application

Activity 1

Examination Procedure	Cranial Nerve Tested
Whisper test	CN VIII
Patient sticking out tongue and moving it from side to side	CN XII
Taste test with sugar, salt, and lemon	CN VII (anterior), CN IX (posterior)
Visual acuity	CN II
Patient puffing out cheeks and showing teeth	CN VII
Patient shrugging shoulders against examiner's hands	CN XI
Smell test with coffee, orange, and cloves	CN I
Eyes constricting and dilating in response to light	CN III
Patient clenching teeth (temporal muscles contracted)	CN V

Activity 2

Age of Infant	Observed Response	Name of Reflex	Expected/Unexpected
8 months	The infant abducts and extends arms and legs in response to sudden movement of head and trunk backward. The arms then adduct in an embracing motion followed by relaxation.	Moro	Unexpected; this should disappear by 6 months of age.
2 months	The infant demonstrates a strong grasp of the examiner's finger when it is placed in the infant's palm.	Palmar grasp	Expected; this should disappear by 3 months.
4 months	When held in an upright position with soles of the feet touching the surface of a table, the infant flexes legs upward in a curled position and holds them there.	Stepping	Unexpected; although the age is appropriate, the expected observed response is an alternating flexion and extension of the legs.
6 months	In a suspended head-first prone position, the infant extends arms and legs.	Parachute	Expected; this should never disappear.

Copyright © 2003, Mosby, Inc. All rights reserved.

Case Study

1. Data deviating from normal: Patient has been diagnosed with CVA. He had headache preceding incident. Patient's history includes inability to talk. He has left-sided paresis. He requires assistance for mobility. Patient avoids eye contact and cries.
2. Ask Mr. Thomas whether he feels he can swallow normally. Ask him whether he has any pain or discomfort. Ask Mrs. Thomas about medical and family history. Ask about medications Mr. Thomas may be currently taking. Ask Mrs. Thomas whether her husband lost consciousness or had a seizure with this incident.
3. Assess gag reflex. Test reflexes (deep tendon). Assess for drooling.
4. Patient has weakness to one side of his body, which affects nearly all aspects of functional abilities. He has problems with communication, nutrition, and mobility as well.

Critical Thinking

1. Kevin's findings are invalid because he did not adjust his tool to determine two-point discrimination. Different body surfaces have varying sensitivity; depending on what body surface is being tested, the distance between two points on tool must be adjusted. For instance, on the fingertips, the minimal distance for the two points is 2.8 mm. On the chest and forearms, the minimal distance is 40 mm. Most body surfaces are not able to detect one-point versus two-point at 1 inch (2.5 mm) apart.
2. The frontal lobe is the primary motor cortex; thus, an infarction in this area will affect motor function primarily on the opposite side of the lesion. Because the patient has a left infarction, he will be affected on the right side. Additionally, if Broca's area is affected, the motor dysfunction will affect this patient's ability to form words.

CHAPTER 22

Content Review

Multiple Choice

1. a
2. c
3. b
4. d
5. a
6. d
7. c
8. c
9. b
10. a
11. d
12. c

Terminology Review

Matching

13. f
14. j
15. h
16. e
17. k
18. m
19. b, c
20. g

Copyright © 2003, Mosby, Inc. All rights reserved.

21. a
22. l
23. d, e
24. m
25. j
26. i
27. m
28. f
29. j
30. m

Concepts Application

Activity 1

Examination Area	Body Systems Examined
Upper extremities	Integumentary, cardiovascular, respiratory, lymphatic, musculoskeletal, neurologic
Anterior chest	Integumentary, cardiovascular, respiratory, lymphatic, musculoskeletal, breasts/axillae
Abdomen	Integumentary, gastrointestinal, cardiovascular, musculoskeletal, lymphatic, neurologic
Head and neck	Integumentary, lymphatic, neurologic, musculoskeletal, visual, auditory, nose/paranasal, mouth/oropharynx

Activity 2

Patient Position	Examination Procedures to Be Included
Sitting with gown on	Head and face, eyes, ears, nose, mouth/pharynx, neck, upper extremities, skin
Sitting with back exposed	Skin, back, chest, lungs
Sitting with anterior chest exposed	Chest, lungs, heart
Reclining at a 45-degree angle	Chest, neck (jugular venous pulsations)
Supine with chest exposed	Heart, breast
Supine with abdomen exposed	Abdomen—auscultation, palpation, reflexes, muscles
Supine with legs exposed	Vascular (pulses, warmth, edema), skin, musculoskeletal

Critical Thinking

1. The most significant modification necessary with this examination is communication. It is vital that the examiner explain what is to be done—and how. Obviously, visual acuity examination will not be necessary, but inspection of the eyes is still applicable.
2. The examiner must maintain composure and express confidence. It is extremely important to identify this patient's concerns and needs through active listening and therapeutic discussion. It is important to be as precise as possible and to set limits as appropriate.

Copyright © 2003, Mosby, Inc. All rights reserved.

CHAPTER 23

Content Review Questions

Multiple Choice

1. b
2. d
3. d
4. a
5. b
6. d
7. c
8. a

Terminology Review

9. false positive
10. specificity
11. true negative
12. negative predictive value
13. Bayes' formula
14. sensitivity
15. true positive
16. false negative
17. positive predictive value

Concepts Application

Activity 1

Symptoms	Body Systems That Might Be Involved
Chest pain	Cardiovascular, pulmonary, musculoskeletal
Headaches	Neurologic, cardiovascular, visual, auditory
Abdominal pain	Cardiovascular, gastrointestinal, urinary
Pain in the legs	Musculoskeletal, neurologic, integumentary, cardiovascular

Activity 2

Examination Findings	Possible Problems
54-year-old female with jaundice, abdominal pain, nausea, weight loss. Has pain to abdominal palpation; positive bowel sounds. Liver slightly enlarged; admits to alcohol use.	Cholecystitis, hepatitis, pancreatitis, cirrhosis, hepatic malignancy
66-year-old male with chief complaint of breathing difficulty. Has increased respiratory rate, low-grade fever, rales, productive cough; increased tactile fremitus bilaterally.	Pneumonia, pulmonary edema, empyema
13-week-old infant girl with fever, irritability, poor eating. Infant is dehydrated and has a temperature of 103.7° F; abdomen soft.	Otitis media, upper respiratory infection, gastroenteritis
19-year-old female college student with chief complaint of pain when urinating. Describes frequency and urgency. Patient has temperature of 100.4° F; Has constant pain in pelvic area; positive pain with fist percussion over left flank.	Urinary tract infection, pyelonephritis, sexually transmitted disease

Copyright © 2003, Mosby, Inc. All rights reserved.

CHAPTER 24

Content Review Questions

Multiple Choice

1. a
2. d
3. c
4. b
5. d
6. b
7. d
8. a
9. c
10. d

Terminology Review

11. subjective
12. chief complaint
13. SOAP
14. illustration
15. Uniform Dental Recording System
16. objective
17. incremental grading
18. POMR
19. health history
20. physical examination

Concepts Application

Problem #	Onset	Problem	Date Resolved
1	June 1998	Low back pain	
2	1977	IDDM—poor control	
3	May 1997	Cholecystitis	
4	1997	Family history ASHD	
5		Family history CRF	

Copyright © 2003, Mosby, Inc. All rights reserved.

Case Study

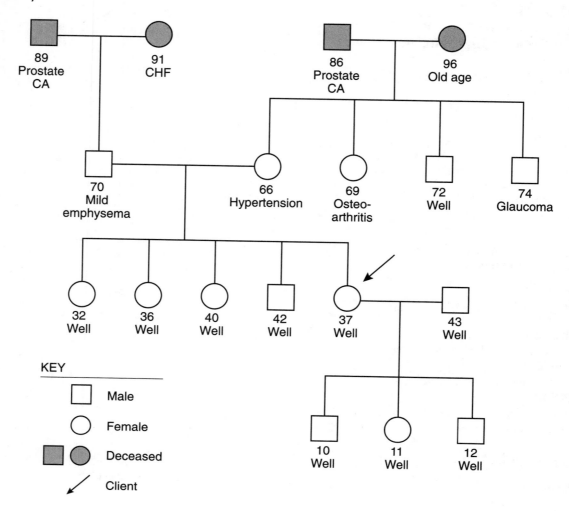

KEY

☐ Male

○ Female

▨ ◗ Deceased

↙ Client

Critical Thinking

1. "OLDCARTS" refers to the following: O = onset of symptom; L = location of the symptom; D = duration of the symptom; C = character of the symptom; A = aggravating/associated factors of the symptom; R = relieving factors; T = temporal factors; S = severity of the symptoms.
2. Organs, masses, and lesions should be documented based on the following characteristics: texture or consistency; size; shape, or configuration; mobility; tenderness; induration; heat; color; location; and other characteristics such as bleeding, discharge, scarring, etc.

CHAPTER 25

Content Review Questions

Multiple Choice

1. a
2. c
3. b
4. c

Copyright © 2003, Mosby, Inc. All rights reserved.

5. a
6. d
7. d
8. a
9. c
10. c
11. b
12. d
13. d
14. b
15. c

Terminology Review

Matching

16. b and e
17. d
18. a and f
19. c
20. f
21. b

Concepts Application

1. primary
2. secondary
3. secondary
4. primary
5. secondary
6. secondary
7. primary
8. primary
9. secondary
10. secondary
11. primary

Case Study

1. Primary assessment findings
   A: Has open airway; is moving air and is able to speak.
   B: Respiratory distress; dyspnea with nasal flaring.
   C: Circulation—has some cyanosis around lips; should palpate pulses.
   D: Is awake and alert, but hypoxic and anxious.
   E: Exposure—no obvious signs of trauma; remove clothing for further assessment.
2. Administration of oxygen
3. Vital signs
4. Primary data deviating from normal include the respiratory data, dyspnea with bloody sputum, and the blood gas findings. His neurologic/mental status suggests hypoxia. Significant from the history is the fact that he is 2 weeks post-op with knee surgery.
5. The most serious concern to continue to monitor for (and treat) is the respiratory status. A priority would be to manage airway and provide ventilatory assistance since his labs indicate he does not have adequate ventilation. A chest x-ray would be helpful.
6. This young man is in serious trouble and if the respiratory status does not improve, death may follow. Initial data suggests an acute pulmonary embolus. Another problem to rule out is drug overdose.

Copyright © 2003, Mosby, Inc. All rights reserved.

Critical Thinking

1. Score = 18. According to the scale, the higher the score, the more likely the child is ill—particularly if the score is greater than 10. Based on his symptoms, this child has significant dehydration.
2. a. Burns and being in a house fire should immediately alert any health care provider to the possibilities of smoke, heat, and/or chemical inhalation. Injuries to the respiratory system may be the most significant injury they suffer.
   b. The examiner must remember that young children and infants have small nasal and oral airway passages; a shorter, narrower trachea; and a short neck. The larynx is higher and more anterior as well. These differences will affect airway management. Second, children have a large body surface area. Children who have suffered burns to the skin are even more susceptible to fluid losses, hypothermia, and infection than are adults.

Copyright © 2003, Mosby, Inc. All rights reserved.